ginkgo biloba

tincture

roots

Healing

Floral remedies

Shiitake

plants

St John's wort

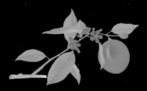

Marie Borrel

CASSELL&CO

2,000

The number of cups of tea that an English person drinks each year. A Frenchman drinks on average 75 to 80. ▶ 76

The Amazonian *Tepuis*, the sacred mountains of the Indians, have only been discovered recently, some of them less than 50 years ago. **9,400** different species of vegetation have been identified there — 40% of which are unknown elsewhere on the planet. ▶ 48

*To date, less than **10**% of known plants have been the subject of serious study.* ▶ 44

*Chinese herbal medicine makes use of more than **20,000** plants.* ▶ 25

St John's wort: a natural antidepressant

From 1997 to 1998 the sales of the natural antidepressant St John's wort increased a hundred-fold in the United States. Secondary effects occur in only **19.8 %** *of cases of people taking it, compared with* **52.8 %** *of those taking chemical antidepressants.*

80 % *of depressed patients who are treated with St John's wort show a marked improvement in only* **4** *weeks.*

 82

Essential oils have a multitude of **properties**: **antiviral**, **antibiotic**, **anti-inflammatory**, **diuretic**, **digestive**, **analgesic**, **tonic**, **laxative**, **sedative**, **expectorant**, anti-rheumatic and calming; they heal wounds, reduce fever and dilate or constrict blood vessels. ▶ 88

Herbalism is not a 'soft' option. Although the ingredients are natural, they can be toxic and therefore dangerous.

Indian herbalism uses more than 3,000 plants, some of which are known to the West, but others not.

Herbalism is the oldest medicine in the world.

Plant hormones are the latest discovery in the modern world of herbalism.

3/4

of the medicines that from plants. 86

The most insignificant blade of grass could well be concealing the gift of healing, containing a property that could form the basis for a powerful new drug.

 47

Observation of the plant kingdom gave rise to one of the most famous medicines on the planet: aspirin.

 17

Herbal medicine is not only a method of healing, it is also a form of philosophy, a particular way of looking at the world.

 34

The depths of tropical forests represent an immense natural greenhouse full of unknown plants. It is here that scientists hope to discover new medicines capable of treating diseases that are currently incurable.

▷ 15

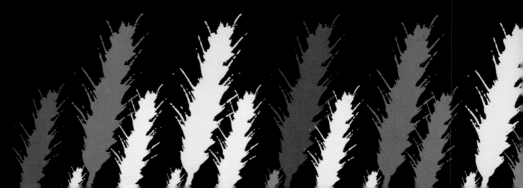

we use in the western world come

Instead of hunting blindly in this immense reservoir of potential new drugs and cures, laboratories have joined forces with anthropologists who study the use of plants by native peoples, and this often throws up the first clues.

 44

Scientific experiments often confirm the wisdom of traditional practices.

 17

The World Health Organisation is putting pressure on governments to encourage the use of herbal medicine so that the knowledge passed on by word of mouth is not lost.

 34

Certain plants contain over 10,000 different molecules. It has taken the Earth more than 4.5 billion years to produce such riches and diversity.

47

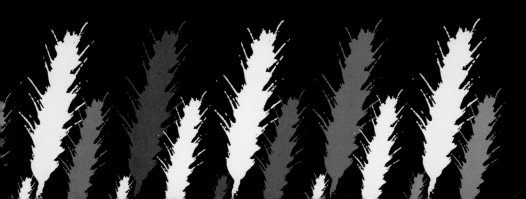

In the Chinese herbal tradition each plant is associated with one of five fundamental flavours: acid, bitter, sweet, spicy and salty. In the West we categorise plants as either stimulating or calming; in Asia this is known as yin and yang.

In China plants are yin or yang according to the energy that they produce.

The Shaman is the guardian
of the sacred nature of plants.
Not everybody can be a Shaman;
he has to be chosen by the spirits
during a dream or a vision.

According to the results of experiments carried out on mice by the University of New Jersey and the Japanese National Cancer Research Institute, the daily consumption of green tea would halt the growth of **87%** of skin cancers, **58%** of stomach cancers and **56%** of lung cancers. 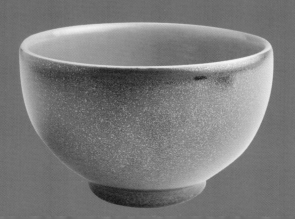 76

'Many plants have healing properties. The ones that I am looking for are the real healing plants, whose work is not to alleviate suffering but to cure and bring the body and the mind back to health.'

Edward Bach

43

From one end of the planet to the other, plants have been attributed with the same powers.

28

Hawthorn, camomile, lavender, marjoram, lemon balm, passion flower, lime tree blossom and valerian are all known for their abilities to reduce stress.

80

Tibetan remedies include dozens of ingredients: plants, minerals and even precious metals.

 31

Each part of the plant can be put to good use; roots, bark, stems, leaves, buds and flowers... Each part is like a small factory producing biologically active molecules.

72

According to the World Health Organisation, about two thirds of the world's population use plants for healing.

 15

8,750
species of tropical trees are currently threatened with extinction.

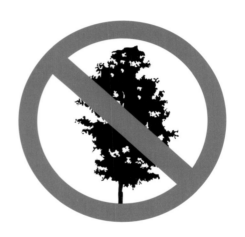

5,000 sq m
of tropical and equatorial forest are disappearing every second.

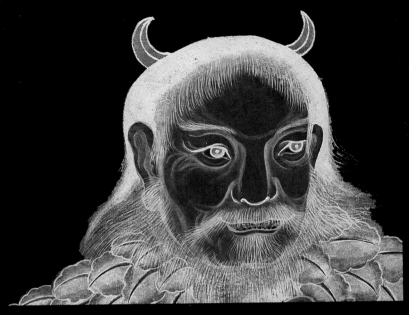

DISCOVER

THE WORLD HISTORY OF HERBALISM AND HEALING PLANTS FROM PREHISTORY TO THE PRESENT DAY: CHINESE MEDICINE AND PLANT ENERGY. THE SHAMAN TRADITION. AYURVEDIC MEDICINE. WESTERN MEDICINE. A LOOK AT CURRENT RESEARCH AND THE MEDICINE OF TOMORROW.

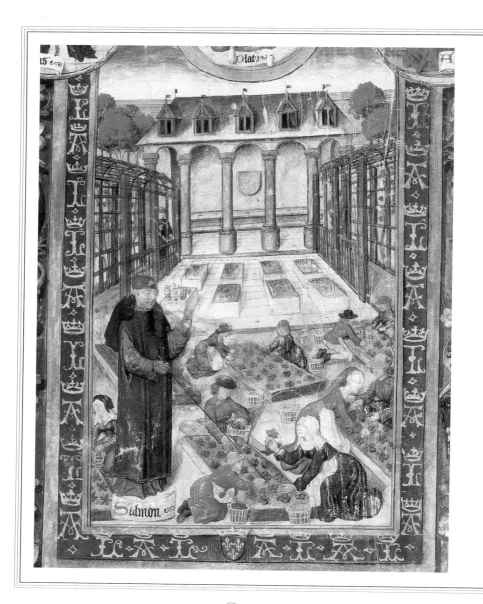

Herbal medicine, or phytotherapy (from the Greek 'phyton' meaning plant) is certainly the oldest form of medicine in the world. Its origins are lost in the distant mists of the prehistoric past. The majority of today's medicines are still derived from plants, whether they contain plant extracts or are created using vegetable molecules as the basis for chemical combinations. However, following the discovery and success of several fundamental medicines, such as sulphonamides in 1908 and antibiotics in 1929, the drugs that stem the spread of certain bacteria, plants lost some of their attraction. Many people came to view their medicinal use as a dubious part of our folklore, and much of the medical world and its patients turned away from them in favour of what science had to offer.

THE CHANGING FACE OF WESTERN HERBAL MEDICINE

In recent years, the image of herbal medicine has undergone a rapid metamorphosis, moving from the dusty herbalist's dispensary to the modern chemist and whole food shop. The apothecaries of the Renaissance stored the powders that they made from medicinal plants in glass bottles. These bottles were labelled with vaguely magical sounding Latin names and sold by weight in little grey or brown paper packets. Today, herbal cures are sold in the same shapes and forms as chemical medicines: in capsules, creams or drops.

A MEDIEVAL HERB GARDEN

Gardens dedicated to the cultivation of medicinal plants were common throughout Europe for many centuries (French manuscript, 15th century).

In countries such as China the traditional knowledge of herbal medicine has been enriched over the centuries and preserved almost intact, despite the fact that Traditional Chinese Medicine was officially abolished in China in 1929. Ironically, it was during this period of decline that Chinese medicine found its way to the West.

In today's world, the two approaches to medicine are becoming less distinct as scientists are looking increasingly to the immense reservoir of unknown plants in the depths of tropical forests, where they hope to find new medicines capable of treating currently incurable diseases.

MEDICINAL PLANTS

The combined interests of two scientists, a French pharmacist, Pierre Joseph Leroux (1795–1870) and a Swiss chemist called Löwig in the medicinal use of plants led to the discovery of one of the most important drugs in the world. Leroux was particularly interested in the bark of the willow tree and in 1827 he discovered that it contained a substance called salicin, which was capable of reducing pain, soothing inflammation and lowering fever. Löwig, meanwhile, was carrying out experiments on the plant known as meadowsweet and in 1840 he discovered that it contained a similar substance to that found in the willow tree, salicylic acid. The combination of their work

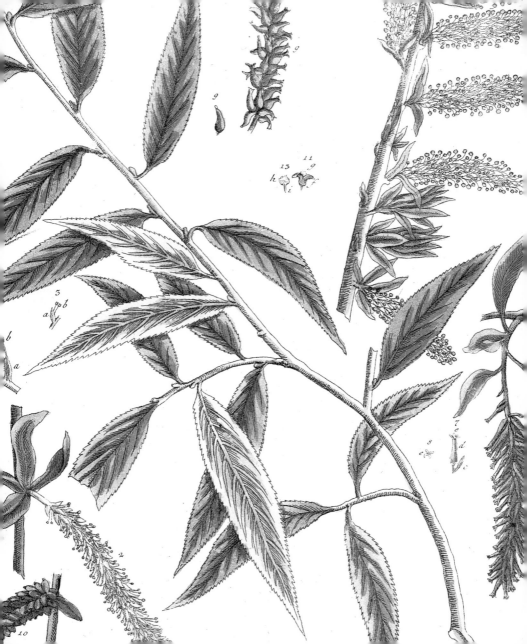

resulted several years later in the production of acetylsalicylic acid, commonly known as aspirin. It is often the case that scientific experiments confirm the wisdom of traditional practices. Quinine, the medicine derived from the bark of the cinchona tree, is a good example. Both the medicine and the extract from the plant itself can be used to calm the violent shaking caused by malarial fevers. Digitalin, which is made from digitalis (the foxglove), is used in treating heart disease.

THE COMPLEXITY OF LIVING PLANTS AND THEIR CONTRIBUTION TO HEALTH

To say that plants are 'complex' means that scientists are not always able to unravel all of their secrets. Molecules extracted from plants often have a dramatic effect on the human body. Inside the plant, a multitude of active ingredients are constantly interacting to heal and, simultaneously, to moderate any side effects on the body. The bark of the willow tree, mentioned previously, is a fine example of this process. It contains salicins that the body transforms into salicylic acid, an analgesic, anti-inflammatory, febrifuge. Unlike manufactured aspirin, which has similar properties, the plant does not have anticoagulant properties. This means that people who suffer from intestinal bleeding can take it without dangerous effects. Meadowsweet, another plant previously mentioned, does not contain gastric acid. This makes it suitable for people who suffer from heartburn or stomach ulcers. A study on rats has even shown that the meadowsweet flower can prevent gastric ulcers from developing. Some pharmacologists believe that the complexity of plants prevents germs (e.g. microbes and bacteria) from adapting and becoming resistant to treatments, which is the converse of what happens with conventional medicine. Thus, quinine has gradually lost its efficacy as a drug, whilst the original plant has kept its healing properties, even though its effect is more modest. Finally, certain plants possess certain properties that resist all analysis. The oil from the leaves of the eucalyptus tree, for example, is well known for its healing action. The molecule responsible for this, eucalyptol, has long been identified and used in the treatment of respiratory diseases. However, this part of the plant also possesses a hypoglycaemic effect that makes it useful in regulating diabetes. Nobody has yet discovered which particular substance is responsible for this action, although it is probably a combination of substances that act simultaneously to reduce the sugar level in the blood, a process known as synergy.

THE WILLOW

Its healing properties have been known for a long time. Twenty-five centuries ago, Hippocrates recommended a herbal tea made with willow leaves to relieve pain and fever.

STRONG PLANTS AND GENTLE PLANTS

Herbal practitioners make a distinction between two sorts of plants: 'strong' plants and 'gentle' plants. Strong plants contain a powerful, dominant substance that has an indisputable effect either on the pathology of a disease or on a precise area or organ of the body. These plants are of particular interest to laboratories as they can either use plant extracts where the active ingredient is produced as a concentrate, or they can produce medicines containing molecules which have come from the active ingredients and have a more precise effect. The first process is known as extraction phytotherapy and the second as phytochemistry.

Gentle plants, on the other hand, are more difficult to break down as they contain numerous substances that act together without any particular one being dominant. Their action depends on global synergy, for this reason they are chiefly of interest to practitioners of traditional herbalism, who tend to make use of the whole plant.

Phytotherapy has played a large part in the growing popularity of alternative or 'gentle' medicine, however, the term 'gentle' is something of a misnomer as this type of treatment is not without its dangers. Gentleness is relative, after all. Certain plants can be harmful to humans and need to be handled with care, particularly those containing actual poisons. Yarrow, for

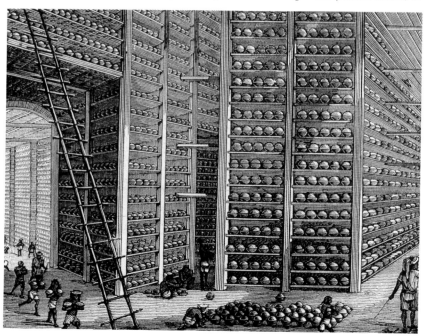

example, is valued for its action on colds and influenza. It can, however, cause severe allergic skin rashes, and prolonged use can increase the skin's photo-sensitivity.

Present-day 'recreational' drugs, both soft and hard, are for the main part derived from plant substances. Heroin is extracted from the poppy, cocaine from the cocoa plant and even tobacco and alcohol both originate from leaves, fruit and cereals. However, all these plants possess healing powers as well – this is particularly true of cannabis.

A serious attempt is being made to evaluate the therapeutic value of cannabis through an ongoing research project in Great Britain involving approximately a million patients. The components of the plant act mainly on the brain, reducing certain types of pain (migraine, rheumatism, pain caused by cancer or multiple sclerosis), lowering blood-pressure in the eye (treating glaucoma) and stimulating the appetite (important for old people who cannot eat properly and those suffering with AIDS). These studies do not aim to legalise cannabis, but to recognise it as a positive source of healing, an aspect of the plant that has been overshadowed by its abuse. Although they have a wealth of healing properties, the complexity of plants means that they also have another, more ambiguous side to them. The negative effects of cannabis are a good example, these include its influence on the reflexes and the effect it has on heartbeat and blood-pressure, causing blackouts and neural changes when large doses are taken. It is important to remember that the sensible use of healing plants is a completely different issue to that of legalisation.

THE MANUFACTURE OF OPIUM AT PATNA IN INDIA

In the East, the use of opium is widespread and opium dens are common. In medicine, this drug is used for its calming and soothing properties (Engraving, 19th century).

WHEN DID MAN FIRST START USING PLANTS FOR MEDICINAL PURPOSES?

Prehistoric man learnt to put meat on a bed of wild mint, basil or rosemary to improve its keeping qualities and slow down deterioration. In the same way, he probably noticed that aromatic plants alleviated the illnesses resulting from eating rotten meat. All we know about the medical practices of prehistoric man comes from scraps of evidence found on the floors of prehistoric caves and shelters. To obtain a more precise picture of the medicinal use of plants, we need to look at historical evidence dating from several thousand years later. The Egyptians left behind them numerous papyri that describe the practice of medicine.

LESSONS TO BE DRAWN FROM EGYPTIAN PAPYRI

Plants were at the heart of healing in ancient Egypt. The Egyptians knew how to extract essential oils from aromatic plants to make precious ointments. They made wide use of barley, hops, aloe, thyme and fenugreek to stop bleeding, heal wounds and fractures and to reduce fever. They even filled decaying teeth with plant resins. This natural stock of plants was deployed within the framework of magic and the gods.

In Egypt, both visible and invisible causes were attributed to diseases. The invisible ones were understood to come from a finely balanced interplay between good and evil and between order and disorder in the world. A whole host of Egyptian gods was responsible for this universal order, including Horus, guardian of health; Thoth, master of medicine and magic; Isis, goddess of fertility; Sekhmet, who unleashed diseases and epidemics when she was angry. Imhotep, the sage and advisor to the pharaoh Zoser (around 2800 BC) laid the foundations of a new medicine and was venerated as a healer god. This explains why the priest-doctors intoned magic formulae and ritual incantations aimed at restoring the broken order at the same time as they dispensed their herbal remedies. This backdrop of magic did not prevent Egyptian healers from perfecting complex formulae, the efficacy of which continues to astonish scientists who analyse samples found in the tombs of the pharaohs.

HORUS

This god of Egyptian mythology, represented by a man with the head of a falcon, was regarded as the guardian of health (Wooden plaque, 900 BC).

HIPPOCRATES AND GALEN: PRECURSORS OF MODERN MEDICINE

The Greek doctor Hippocrates, born on the small island of Cos in about 460 BC, has had a considerable influence on Western medicine and is regarded as the father of modern medical practice. He was the first doctor to establish a code of ethics for the medical profession and to advocate meticulous observation of the facts before suggesting even the slightest of theories, thus closing the door on the sometimes fantastic speculations of his predecessors. He laid the foundations for the first medical clinics, making the questioning of patients as well as listening to their chests an indispensable part of the diagnosis. On top of this, he was particularly interested in the patient's hygiene and nutrition and frequently prescribed plant-based remedies to cure their ills. The tradition of using plants in the process of healing was greatly enriched over many centuries in which observations and discoveries were transmitted by word of mouth from one generation to the next. By the time of Hippocrates, the European herbal tradition had already absorbed ideas from Assyria and India. Plants were mixed to create potions and ointments to which animal or mineral substances were sometimes added to thicken them. The oldest illustrated botanical manuscripts date from the first century AD: *De Materia Medica by Dioscorides* (c.40–c.90) and *Codex Anicae Julianae*, a Byzantine version of Dioscorides' text. The plants were described and drawn, and both their healing and harmful properties were noted. These manuscripts changed the way in which knowledge about plants was transmitted forever.

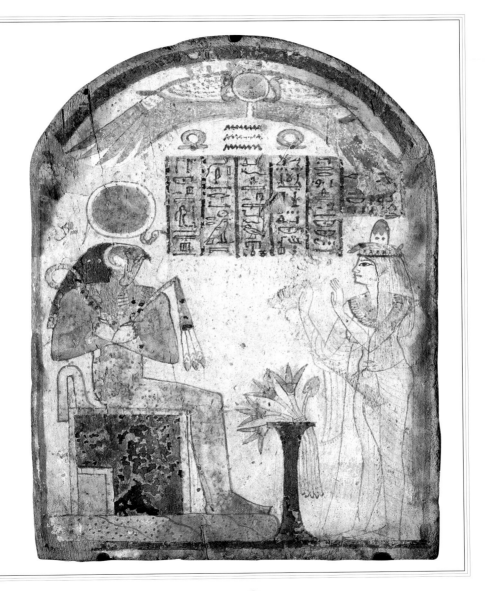

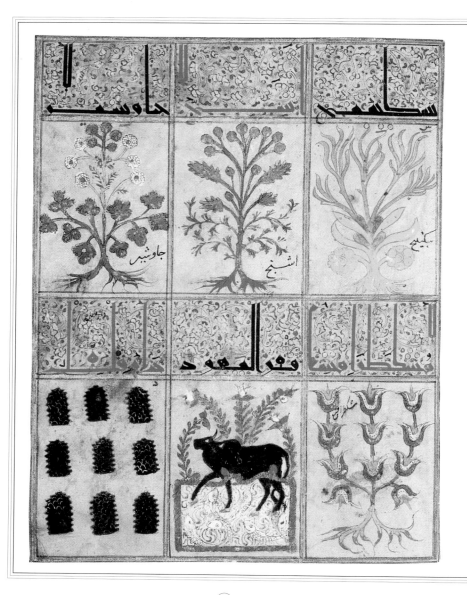

Diocles of Caryste, a follower of Hippocrates, drew up the first herbal (a list of plants and their uses) known to the Western world during the fourth century, and from then onwards the body of knowledge about plants began to take on a more definitive structure.

At the beginning of the 11th century AD, Claudius Galenus was born at Pergamum. This Greek doctor made a significant contribution to the history of medicine, although he was not well liked by his contemporaries who found him vindictive and arrogant. A follower of Hippocrates, he continued the practice of rigorous observation of his patients and made progress in the area of anatomy by studying the physique of gladiators and dissecting animals. Like Hippocrates, he also used plants in his treatments. He became famous for his meticulous study of plants and their preparation for medicinal purposes, a method which is still known as Galenic pharmacy and is used by many modern laboratories to prepare medicinal plants for sale.

COLD CREAM

It is to Claudius Galenus that we owe the recipe for cold cream composed of no less than seventy-four ingredients. This remedy was prescribed mainly to cure poisonings (Arabian book, 1199).

ANCIENT CHINA: THE ENERGY SIGNATURES OF PLANTS

On the other side of the globe during this same period the Chinese were also experimenting with the healing properties of plants. Their observations resulted in an entirely different set of medical theories. Chinese medicine is one of the oldest in the world, with some texts dating back to before 2500 BC. It is based wholly upon a notion that is unknown to Western science, that of energy.

In Traditional Chinese Medicine, illness is seen as a sign of disharmony within the patient. The task of the Chinese practitioner is to restore the harmony and balance of the body, enabling its natural healing mechanisms to work more efficiently. Herbs are a vital part of the treatment.

The theory of opposites is central to Chinese thought. Energy has twin poles: *yin* and *yang*. Everything that is fluid, cold, wet, passive, dark, and internal is *yin* in character, as are all things that are feminine in nature such as the moon, night, water and winter. Everything that is solid, warm, bright, active and external is *yang* in character as are all things masculine in nature such as the sun, fire and summer. *Yin* and *yang* are two principles inherent throughout nature. The first represents rest and the second activity. Like all opposites, they both complement and oppose each other. The principal symbolic *yin/yang* couple is that of the Earth and the sky: the Earth is solid, heavy, dense and obscure whereas the sky is inconstant, subtle, light, translucent and bright. In all things living, both human and animal, the male/female couple is the incarnation of this dynamic.

Inside the body, the same scenario is played out: when an organ becomes too yin, there is a reduction in the physiological metabolism (slowing down of heartbeat and digestion, feelings

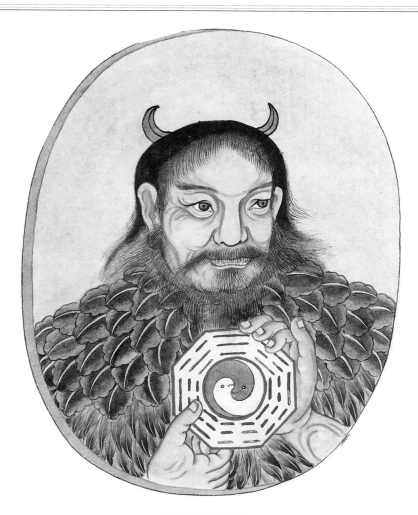

THE EMPEROR FOU-HI

Wearing a costume of leaves, Fou-Hi holds in his hands both yin and yang
(Water-colour taken from a pen-ts'ao, a book of medicinal plants, end of 18th – beginning of 19th century).

of cold and signs of pallor). Conversely, if part of the body becomes too *yang*, there is an acceleration of the physiological metabolism (increased heartbeat, feelings of warmth, physical and mental hyperactivity). The two opposing elements should remain balanced, as a good balance is believed to sustain life and ensure good health.

The life energy which runs through the human body nourishes it and keeps it alive; it circulates through the body along channels called meridians. If this circulation is harmonious, fluid and regular the individual is in good health. But if it accumulates in certain places and is missing in others, then adverse symptoms appear. To regulate this circulation the Chinese have several tools at their disposal: meditation, nutrition, acupuncture and above all plants. The Chinese pharmacopoeia (book of plants) contains more than 20,000 entries! In China, plants are primarily administered in their natural form. Chinese doctors prescribe mixtures of dried plants (leaves, flowers, stalks and roots) that pharmacists make up for the patient, these are most commonly used as decoctions or essences. Dried plant extracts are also available and are sold in the form of powder, pills or tablets and made up according to well-known formulae.

SUBTLE INTERPLAY: HOW TO FIND A PLANT CAPABLE OF RESTORING THE ENERGY BALANCE

In Chinese medicine, plants are categorised primarily by the type of energy that they dispense, either *yin* or *yang*. A *yin* plant has dispersal qualities, such as clearing out, calming, sleep-inducing and cooling down; it slows down the reactions of an organism. It is therefore used for calming the excesses of *yang*. Conversely, a *yang* plant tones and stimulates, encourages secretions, awakens and warms; it accelerates the reactions of the body and is used to calm the excesses of *yin*.

Plants are thus identified and classified according to whether they stimulate or disperse the energy of the main organs – for example the liver, the heart, the spleen, the lungs and the kidneys. Another quality which affects the energy of plants is their capacity to regulate cold and warmth; certain herbal remedies have a warming effect whilst others cool down the body when it becomes too hot. In the same way, some plants soak up excess humidity when there are too many secretions and others moisten an organism which has become too dry.

The last aspect to consider in the categorisation of plants is the different flavours that they possess. In the Chinese tradition, everything that grows on this earth belongs to one of five fundamental flavours: acidic, bitter, sweet, salty or spicy. Each flavour is linked to one of the five main organs: the liver correlates to acidic flavours, the lungs to spicy ones, the spleen to sweet things, the heart to bitter flavours and the kidneys to salty ones. As the Chinese concept of medicine dictates that the condition of these five organs is the key to having a balanced body, an adjustment of flavours or plants is theoretically sufficient to re-establish the balance. Thus, an excess of *yin* in the liver is cured by a *yang* plant with an acidic flavour. If there is too much *yang* in the heart, the doctor will prescribe a *yin* plant with a bitter flavour.

This system of classification allows traditional Chinese doctors to fine-tune the choice of herbal treatment depending on the diagnosis. It would be tempting to find out if this 'energetic' approach could have a bearing on similar applications in the Western world, however the native plants used in the Chinese pharmacopoeia are very different to ours. Nevertheless, some Western doctors who practise Chinese medicine have tried to classify Western healing plants according to the traditional Chinese method.

A BRIDGE BETWEEN EAST AND WEST

In ancient texts of herbal medicine, Western plants were grouped according to five categories that match the Chinese classification. These groups consisted of plants containing organic acids (acidic flavour); those containing alkaloids (bitter flavour); ones containing mucilage and fatty acids (sweet flavour); those containing iron or sulphur (spicy flavour) and plants containing organic salts (salty flavour).

Similarly the Chinese notion of *yin* and *yang* energy is paralleled in Western notions of stimulating plants and sedative plants. There is another possible *yin/yang* system of classification that depends on the effect of plants on the central nervous system. This consists of two branches: the sympathetic nervous system that activates and stimulates the vital functions (the accelerator) and the parasympathetic nervous system that tempers it (the brake). Thus, if a plant stimulates the sympathetic system it is classified as *yang* and if it stimulates the parasympathetic it is classified as *yin*.

THE THREE FLAVOURS

Buddha, Lao-Tseu and Confucius gather around a vinegar pot trying to determine its flavour. The first one finds it bitter, the second sour and the third sweet.

In the light of this classification, all that needs to be done is to compare the usual indications of the plants and their type of energy. Let us take the example of *Anemone pulsatilla*, a *yin* plant with an acidic flavour. In China it is used to calm down excess *yang* in the liver. In the West, it is traditionally used to treat increased heartbeat, neuralgia, migraines, bronchial spasms, allergic rhinitis, painful periods, anxiety and phobias; however, these same symptoms, according to Chinese medicine show an excess of *yang* in the liver.

Another example is camomile. According to Chinese classification, it is a *yang* plant with a sweet flavour. In China it would be used to calm an excess of *yin* in the spleen. In the West, it is used to cure a lack of appetite, chronic stomach pain, fatigue, anaemia, a lack of white blood-cells and an absence of periods. For a Chinese doctor, these symptoms signal an excess

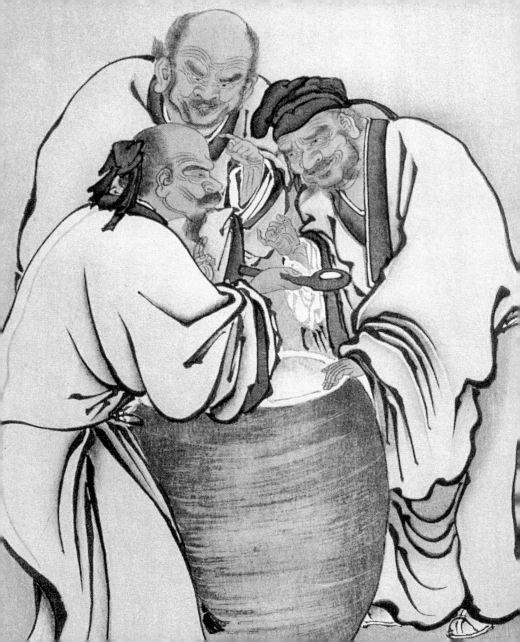

of *yin* in the spleen. It can be argued, therefore, that these two different traditions, separated by several centuries and millions of miles, follow one and the same path. It seems that whatever route men take to unravel the secrets hidden in plants their properties will eventually be revealed.

THE AYURVEDIC TRADITION: PREVENTATIVE AND CURATIVE PRACTICES STILL WIDELY USED IN INDIA

Ayurvedic medicine, the traditional medicine of ancient India, developed between 600 and 100 BC. The word 'Ayurveda' literally means 'the science of life'. One of the early texts of this religion states that 'Everything which is found in the universe can be found in a human being and everything which is in a human being can be found in the universe'. This premise places man at the centre of his environment. It is through this belief that the individual can find a balanced path, because man, like everything that surrounds him, is only one of the many manifestations of primordial energy according to the Ayurvedic tradition.

A CHINESE PHARMACY
The numerous pots and drawers are indispensable for storing the countless remedies drawn from the Chinese pharmacopoeia, which is one of the oldest in the world.

Ayurvedic medicine is not focused solely on healing diseases, its purpose is complete health: physical, emotional, mental and spiritual. To achieve this, the Ayurvedic doctor concentrates on the patient not the disease, using a system of 'constitutions' or 'doshas'. Ayurvedic medicine is used to determine the constitution or body type of an individual. Like homeopathy, it uses 'constitutions' as points of reference. There are three doshas (*vata*, *pitta* and *kapha*) which are present in each living being and when they are perfectly balanced the individual is deemed to be in excellent health. As soon as one of the *doshas* becomes more dominant than the other two, disease can take hold.

The use of plants is omnipresent in traditional Indian medicine and they are administered according to precise rules. First of all, the time of day should be taken into consideration – different remedies need to be taken at different times of day. Each hour of the day corresponds to one of five symbolic elements: water, fire, earth, air or ether (the intangible). For example, the hour of Brahman, two hours before sunrise, is considered to be the ideal time for getting up. This hour belongs to the air element when the mind is particularly calm. It is the time of day that stimulates elimination. This means on getting up, it is advisable to drink a glass of water without food, and then to take plants which favour elimination. When the sun rises, the air element gives way to water. When the sun is at its peak, it is the time of fire and energy and this is when toning, energising plants that stimulate deficient organic functions are recommended.

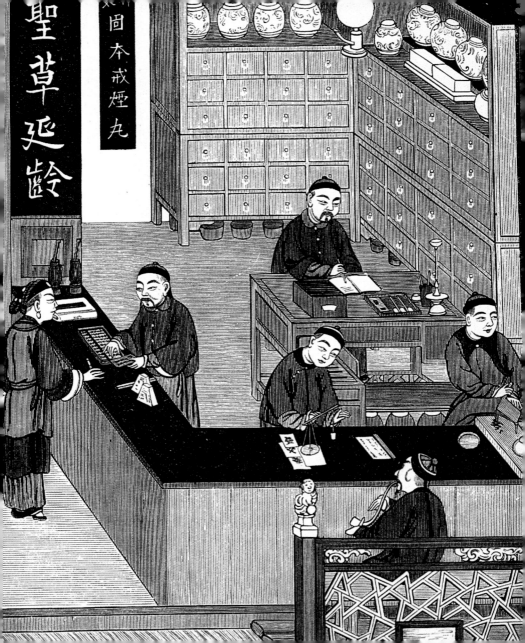

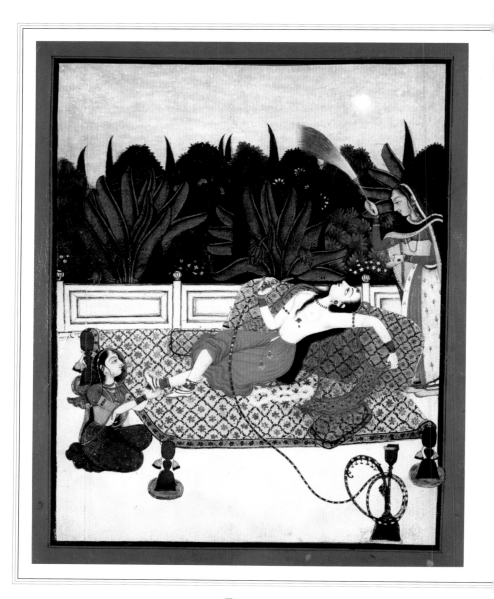

Indian herbalism uses more than 3,000 species of plants, some of which are known in the West (garlic, ginger, saffron and cinnamon) and others which are not commonly known (amalaki, harithaki, neem). According to tradition, these plants act together in different ways depending on their material substance, their flavour (as in Chinese medicine) and the properties that digestion gives to them. In each case, their aim is to bring the doshas back into harmony, as their imbalance is seen to be the cause of the disease.

In the Ayurvedic tradition, plants are prepared in a wider variety of ways than in the Chinese tradition. In India, plant juice (*swaras*), plant mixtures (*kaika*), decoctions (*kashyas*), macerations (*hiema*) and infusions (*phanta*) are used as well as powders and capsules made with mixtures of different plants. One of the flagship remedies of Ayurvedic medicine, *triphala*, is a mixture containing three local plants which simultaneously balance the doshas, regenerate the colon, regularise the digestion and the metabolism and eliminate toxins.

Finally, massage plays an important role in this form of treatment along with nutrition and meditation. Massages are given using plant oils enriched with essences – providing yet another way of benefiting from the healing properties of plants.

MEDICINE FROM THE ROOF OF THE WORLD

On the borders of India, in the high Himalayan plateaux, there is a small, isolated country which has an extraordinary medicinal heritage. Tibetan medicine has drawn its main inspiration from neighbouring India, but over the centuries it has been enriched by influences from China and the Persian Empire, as well as the Shamanic practices of the local population. Out of this crucible has come a powerfully spiritual approach to healing in which plants play a very important role. There is a great diversity of flora on the high plateaux, where plants are less likely to be damaged by harmful pollution. Some of the plants are used in infusions, decoctions and macerations, but the majority are fashioned into small, hand-made pills. Tibetan remedies contain dozens of ingredients including plants, minerals and precious metals. Some pills, for example, contain gold, silver, turquoise or coral mixed with numerous plants; their combined effect is believed to relieve the diseases that spiritual healing has been unable to cure. The nub of Tibetan medicine lies in discovering the true cause of the illness. This can involve delving into the past since, being Buddhists, Tibetans believe in reincarnation. It is not unusual for Tibetans to refer back to a past life to explain a symptom that resists all treatment.

Practically wiped out by the Chinese invasion in 1951, traditional Tibetan medicine was preserved by a few practitioners who jealously guarded their secrets. In fact, it was the

FOOT MASSAGE

Foot massage is very relaxing. In Ayurvedic medicine, plant-based oils are often used in massage.

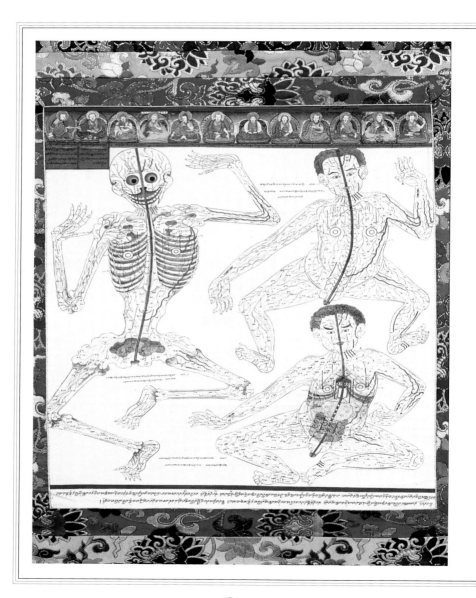

effectiveness of the medicine that ensured its survival. In spite of resistance, the Chinese who were living in Tibet after the invasion had to resort to using the few Tibetan healers that still remained in the country. Tendzin Choedrak, doctor of the Dalai Lama, spent many years locked up in Chinese prisons. Despite his criminal status under Chinese law, he was called upon to cure Chinese high officials, who later authorised him to start researching and collecting traditional medical texts that had survived. Today he lives in the north of India where the exiled Tibetan community continue to make pills from plants using the ingredients prescribed by their ancestors.

TIBETAN MEDICINE

Tibetan medicine has drawn its main inspiration from neighbouring India, but over the centuries it has been enriched by influences from China and Persia as well.

Choedrak still participates every year in medical congresses, where he presents the results of work carried out on plants in the research centre of Dharamsala.

SHAMANISM: THE SPIRIT OF PLANTS

On every continent, ethnic medicines still survive on the fringes of more orthodox approaches. In all these practices, illness is seen as a visual manifestation of a problem in the invisible world, the realm of the spirit. To cure the disease an intercessor capable of communicating with the other world is required; this role is assumed by the witch-doctor or Shaman.

In Shamanic medicine, plants are not used for their physical or chemical healing properties but for their 'spirit', which can intercede on behalf of the patient, or because they help the Shaman to change his state of consciousness in order to enter into communication with the spirits. During ritual ceremonies, hallucinogenic plants are consumed in a symbolic context to help this communication, which is seen as indispensable to healing.

The Shamanic concept of the universe invests everything that exists with a spirit: the Earth, the sun, the stars, stones, animals and plants. These spirits represent the living essence of things and have a life of their own. They can work for the good of man or bring misfortune in the form of bad luck, illness or madness. The Shaman is thus an integral part of this hidden universe.

Plants are used by Shamans in many different ways. The North American Indian Shamans participate in ceremonies in sweat tents. The tent is heated by red-hot stones. The participants sit naked in the tents and allow the perspiration to wash their bodies and souls of all their impurities. Herbs are burnt in the tent and the spirits of the plants are believed to take part in the purification. This cleansing is an indispensable prerequisite for other rituals, which require the participant to present himself to be as innocent as a new-born baby. Plants are either chewed, crushed in a mortar, pulverised and inhaled, or burnt, depending on the area of the country in which the ritual takes place. Sometimes the Shaman heals by chanting the names of plants, but he always respects their sacred character.

This tradition of chanting is still alive in certain countries such as Siberia, despite advances in civilisation, and is transmitted by word of mouth from master to pupil, showing great reverence for the knowledge of their ancestors. Thus, little by little, an extremely rich body of botanical knowledge has developed, to which modern science has turned its attention in the hope of discovering ingredients for new medicines. This source of expertise is considered to be so important that the World Health Organisation has, on numerous occasions, asked governments to encourage the use of traditional medicines, so that this knowledge, preserved only in oral tradition, does not disappear.

MEANWHILE IN EUROPE...

Chinese, Ayurvedic and Shamanic medicine have all developed slowly over the years with each new discovery adding to the traditional body of knowledge without in any way contradicting it. These forms of treatment are not merely methods of healing, they are also philosophies, ways of looking at the world that need to be embraced before using the cures that they afford. Orthodox, Western medicine has evolved in a completely different way. Never have the people in the West lived so long or been so healthy as they are today, and yet, the medical profession has never aroused such doubts or disapproval.

During the Middle Ages medical progress was hindered when the Church forbade the dissection of bodies. Unable to conduct anatomical research, doctors still followed the ancient texts of Hippocrates and Galen. As the centuries passed, a gap opened up between every-day healing practises based on traditional plant remedies and the medical discoveries of a scientific élite. Certain individuals who were interested in the medical use of plants fell somewhere between these two extremes.

THE HEALER

People who are destined to be Shamans are chosen by spirits during dreams or visions. They are then initiated by older Shamans whom they replace (Georges Catlin, The Indians of North America, 1848).

Hildegarde von Bingen is a unique example. One of the greatest monastic figures of the Middle Ages and an extraordinary woman, she was respected for her theological writings, her music and her knowledge of the medicinal uses of plants. Born in 1098 into a rich family in the Mayence region of Germany, she took her vows at the age of 14 and her early vocation sustained her right up until her death at nearly 80 years of age. Throughout her life she had visions, premonitions and apparitions and worked tirelessly to interpret these signs and to convey a meaningful message through her numerous writings. One of her works, entitled *Physica*, was largely dedicated to plants.

Hildegarde von Bingen believed that, exiled from heaven, man had become vulnerable to the forces of nature. Although she saw man as essentially a feeble creature, her belief in God convinced her that everything necessary to cure man's ills could be found in nature. She drew

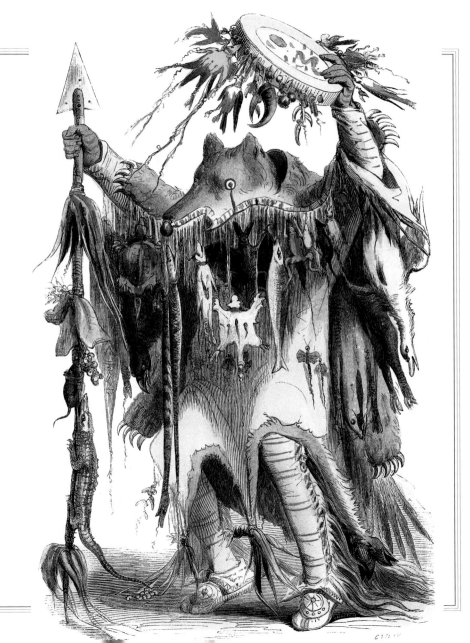

up an impressive list of complex herbal recipes, with strict instructions for preparations, that were religious in essence. These included herbal teas and subtle flower essences as well as recipes for creating vapours and 'packs' to be applied to the body. In her writings she even refers to plants from the Far East, such as galangal, which were still unknown in the West at this time, and her advice on the uses of this plant corresponds completely with what we know about the plant today. In the uncertain medical context of the time, the precision of Hildegarde von Bingen stands alone among those of her contemporaries.

PARACELSUS AND THE THEORY OF SIGNATURES

Three centuries later, in about 1493, Paracelsus was born. This Swiss doctor and alchemist was responsible for a theory that still astonishes scientists today. Paracelsus believed that nature itself provided man with an instruction manual on the use of plants; he thought that it was only necessary to observe the shape, colour and location of plants in order to understand their possible uses.

Once again the willow can be used to illustrate this point. The willow tree grows in damp areas, near ponds and marshes, thus Paracelsus believed that it should be used to cure illnesses caused by similar conditions. He recommended that it be used to ease rheumatism and to lower the temperature, a use which science later confirmed in the production of aspirin, one of the main ingredients of which comes from the willow tree. The autumn crocus (meadow saffron) provides another example. With a bulb resembling a gout-ridden toe, by the same logic, it was thought to cure gout, and sure enough the autumn crocus does possess an active ingredient which relieves attacks of gout. In the same way, rhubarb, still recommended today to encourage the production of bile, possesses a yellow juice resembling bile.

PARACELSUS

Plants 'indicate' their use. 'Everything that nature creates', wrote Paracelsus, is shaped in the image of the property that is associated with it' (Engraving, 16th century).

This blind belief in the existence of a natural order is summed up in the formula *similia similibus curantur* (like cures like), a maxim which forms the basis of the doctrine of signatures. For example, yellow plants, such as the saffron crocus, were used to treat jaundice, and red substances, such as rust or red wine, were thought to be good for 'bloodlessness' or anaemia. Samuel Hahnemann, who perfected *infinitesimal* medicine at the end of the 18th century, also refers to the doctrine of signatures.

HAHNEMANN'S GREAT DISCOVERY

Like Paracelsus and Hildegarde von Bingen, Hahnemann (1755–1843) thought that God, an essentially benign force, had put within man's reach everything that he needed to cure his ills.

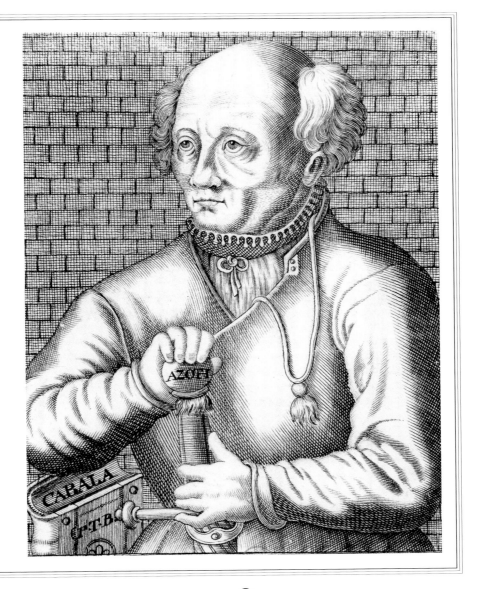

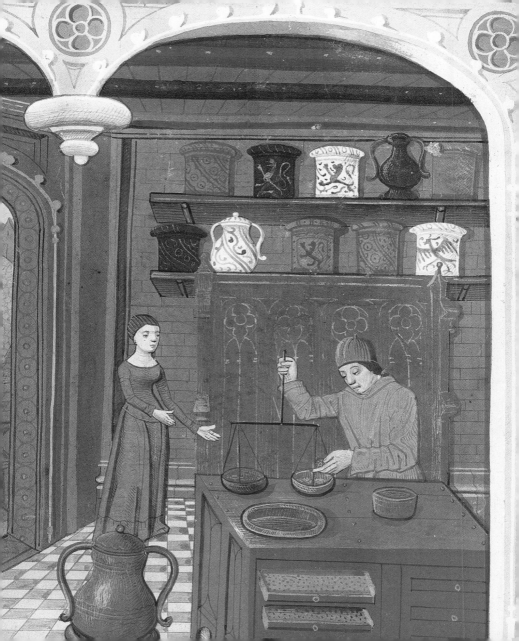

It was up to man, therefore, to discover this hidden knowledge. He wrote the following on the subject: 'There is an important truth that is evident all around us. We cannot believe that God has forgotten to equip us to combat evil. He makes the harvest ripen and the crops grow. Why would he neglect to ensure our health and well-being through the same elements of air, light and water?'

Hahnemann found his path to be a long and painful one. A young, intelligent man living in the German town of Saxe, he had chosen to enter the medical profession at the age of 19. The world of medicine at that time struck him as both obscure and full of charlatans. 'Doctors are strange for they introduce remedies that they are unfamiliar with into bodies that they know even less about', he observed. He was hungry for research, for knowledge and for science.

AN APOTHECARY'S SHOP

From the Middle Ages, plants were sold to be used in the form of teas, infusions and decoctions (15th-century illuminated book).

After years of practising medicine, he still remained dissatisfied by his powerlessness to cure using the means available to him at the time. One day, a child died in his arms. This was one death too many for him. He decided to abandon the practice of medicine until he had found what he was looking for, although he was unsure what this was. To earn a living he started to do translation work and it was whilst translating a passage about the bark of the cinchona tree from an English medical text, that he made a remarkable discovery. At the time, doctors prescribed the bark of the cinchona tree for temperatures and feverishness. Cuellan suggested that the action of the plant was due to its effects on the nerves of the stomach. Hahnemann realised that there was a very simple way of testing whether this was true: 'let a healthy body absorb the remedy and see what happens' he said. The amazing result was that the cinchona bark produced in him the symptoms that it was meant to cure: sweating, trembling and anxiety. Hahnemann realised the importance of his discovery. He saw that a plant that produces symptoms highly similar to those of a disease may also be used to cure it. A splendid illustration of Paracelsus' theory of *similia similibus curantur*.

FROM HOMEOPATHY TO ANTHROPOSOPHY

For many years Hahnemann experimented in this way with all the remedies of the pharmacopoeia of the time, mainly with plants but also with minerals and animal substances, meticulously noting the physical and mental reactions that they caused. The impressive amount of notes that he accumulated served as the basis for a book that was unprecedented in the history of medicine. However, certain substances were so toxic in strong doses that he undertook to reduce them to infinitesimal amounts by diluting them again and again. This process gave birth to the practice of homeopathy, a form of treatment which cures like with like using amounts so small that, according to the laws of physics, there is often nothing left in the remedies. The practice of homeopathy still stirs up the medical fraternity today, divided as they are into its supporters and opponents. The fact remains, however, that this way of healing, although criticised for its lack of scientific rigour, was born in the mind of a man who hungered after science and research. Homeopathy is based on the rigorous observation of the effects of plants on the human body, a task that had never been undertaken with such precision before.

In 1861, more than 20 years after the death of Hahnemann, a man destined to continue his work was born in Hungary. His name was Rudolph Steiner, and he became the creator of anthroposophy, a philosophy that places man at the centre of creation. Anthroposophy has several applications: it provides the basis of a method of teaching, a form of architecture, agriculture and, of course, a form of medicine in which plants play a very important and special part.

Steiner was a fervent admirer of the great German poet Goethe (1749–1832), who published several scientific tracts dedicated to optics, colours and, above all, plants (*The Metamorphosis of Plants*, 1790). At the age of 19 Goethe was saved from serious illness by an alchemic remedy prescribed by an old and very religious doctor. From then on he developed a passion for cures and plants, losing faith in his doctor's knowledge. Goethe felt that it was impossible to study a living organism by isolating it in time and space, as happened when a plant was picked and put into a herbarium (a systematically organised collection of dry plants). He believed that a plant should be observed whilst alive, during its various stages of growth and evolution, a belief which gave birth to his theory of metamorphosis, from which Steiner drew most of his inspiration.

STEINER'S THEORY

An intellectual and a profoundly spiritual person, Steiner regarded man as an entity comprising three parts: the body, the mind and the soul. According to him, man was a summary of nature and the universe, representing the last stage in creation. He carried within him, therefore, the three essential components of nature, mineral, animal and vegetable, added to which was a fourth dimension specific to man, that of conscience. Steiner believed that everything that exists in the world also exists in man, including the plant world and its myriad species. Naturally, Steiner used plants to cure diseases. He regarded plants as men upside down, with their feet in the air and their mental processes buried in the earth. Man functioned on three physical levels: below (the abdominal area) a metabolic centre controlled the vital functions; on top (the brain) a neuro-sensory centre controlled perceptions and thought, and

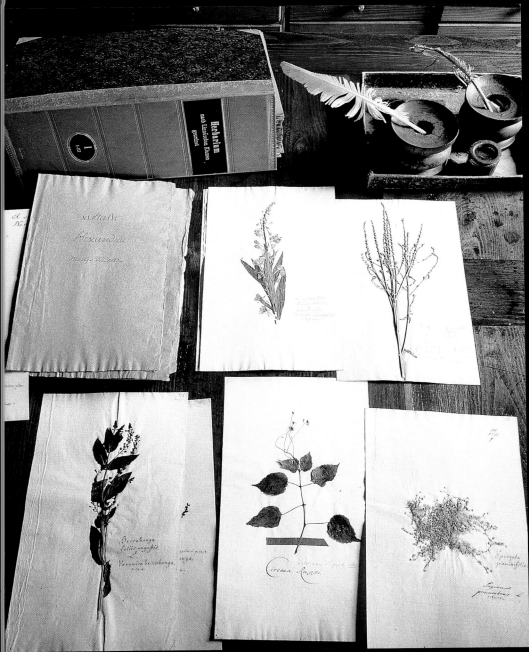

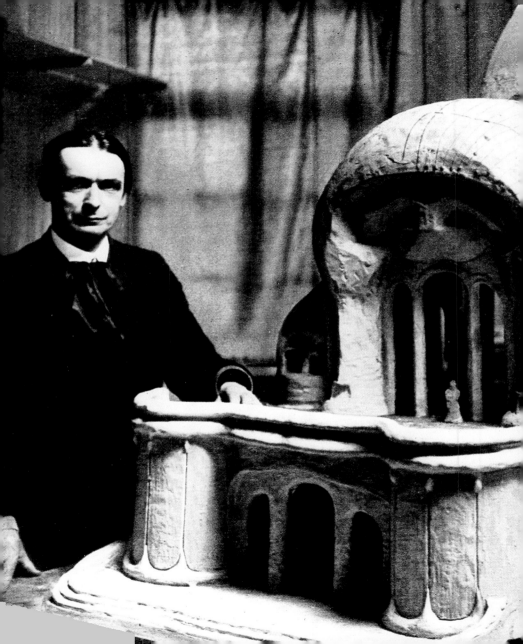

between the two (the thorax) there was a rhythmic centre which linked the top and the bottom. Any imbalance between these areas would result in illness. As far as plants were concerned, their sensorial centre was buried in the earth, and took the form of roots seeking nourishment, whilst the flowers and fruits, centres of intense metabolic activity were situated at the higher level. Between the two, the leaves, with their regular development, represented the rhythmic centre. To cure a patient, Steiner recommended using the part of the plant that corresponded to the area which was causing the patient problems. So, for example, the roots

of *Chamomilla*, camomile, known for its calming properties, are used to balance neuro-sensory activity and its flowers are used to regularise metabolic activity. By observing plants in the same way as Goethe, that is as they developed in their living state, Steiner evaluated their actions. The choice of plant was made according to a principle similar to Paracelsus' doctrine of signatures. An elegant, slender silver birch could not 'behave' in the same way as a stocky, gnarled oak, whilst a fern, which produces lots of leaves and few roots, could not be the same as a bryony which has more roots and few leaves. The last stage of the process is known asdilution. Like Hahnemann, Steiner diluted the basic substances to make their action subtler and to render them more easily accessible to the human body. He even went as far as using the plants themselves in the process of dilution. Instead of artificially mixing a plant and a mineral in the same medicine, he fed the first with the second so that everything would happen naturally. The anthroposophic medicine, *Primula Auro culta*, which brings together gold and primroses to cure heart and circulation problems, stems from this system. To produce this medicine, a primrose root is planted in a mixture of earth and gold and the plant is left to grow for a year before being harvested for the preparation of the medicine.

EDWARD BACH: THE SUBTLE ESSENCE OF FLOWERS

Anthroposophic principles shocked those with more logical minds. The principles seemed to make a mockery of the chemical facts, dismissing them in favour of a more ethereal, spiritual vision of the world and of life itself, which encompassed both men and plants. At the beginning of the 20th century, the ideas of Edward Bach, an English doctor whose main interest was flowers, were even more subtle. Bach was convinced that illnesses had a strong spiritual element and that emotional balance therefore was the best guarantee of health and the first instrument of healing.

A tireless worker, he practised first of all in hospitals before becoming interested in homeopathy. Like all his illustrious predecessors, he was convinced that the solution to man's problems was concealed in nature's hidden depths. He abandoned his medical practice to scour the country-side's natural resources. Gradually, he became convinced that flowers contained the spirit of plants and that the breath, the essence, and all the healing energy of the plant world resided in flowers. He began by making homeopathic dilutions, then he moved on to natural alchemy using moisture and the sun's rays. Collecting the morning dew from petals and making remedies that were intended to harmonise different states of mind and thus restore health.

As public demand reached ever higher levels, he looked for a method of production that was less restrictive than collecting dew. He came up with the idea of leaving the flowers to soak for several hours in spring water, whilst being exposed to the first rays of the sun, in the place where they were growing. He had finally found the simple, natural method that he had been seeking all along; fire, earth and air working together to produce remedies. In this way Bach developed 38 floral remedies, each one corresponding to a state of mind and capable of regularising excesses of anger, timidity or anxiety.

SILENT CONVERSATIONS

These idealistic views of nature may raise a smile, but Bach, Steiner and Hahnemann created methods of healing that, although they have aroused derision in the scientific world, are still in use today. Floral remedies are widely used in Britain, homeopathy is gathering support in Britain and elsewhere in Europe, as are anthroposophic remedies.

The complexity of the plant world and its sense of mystery, have helped to fuel an interest in different forms of herbal medicine in many parts of the Western world today.

There is a school of thought that supports the theory that plants can communicate with one another in a way that humans cannot detect, using chemicals. These messages are said to be numerous and to pass completely unnoticed by our sensory organs which are too rudimentary to grasp them. Plants communicate to protect each other from predators. Poplars, oaks and maples, for example, warn each other when an invasion of predatory insects is approaching by secreting toxic substances that will render them indigestible. Other plants, maize for example, produce cocktails of chemicals that will attract the predators that feed on their parasites, thus disposing of them. The sensitivity of plants never ceases to amaze researchers and new discoveries are being made every day.

BACH'S OFFICE

Doctor Bach created 38 floral remedies. Other scientists all over the world have continued his work.

WESTERN MEDICINES DERIVED FROM TROPICAL FORESTS

Up to now only ten per cent of plant species on this planet have been studied in depth. Rather than searching blindly, Western laboratories have chosen to join forces with

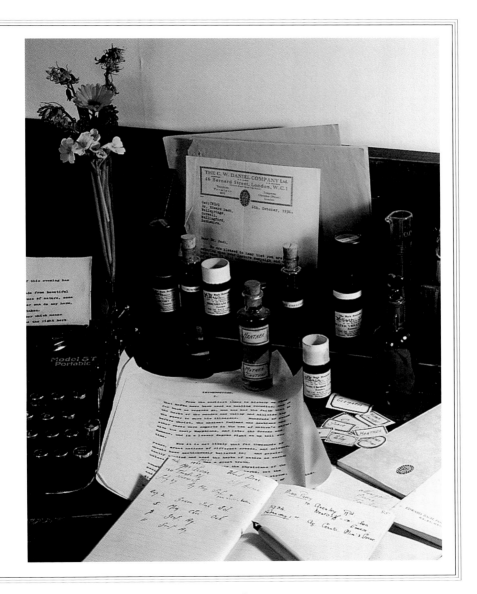

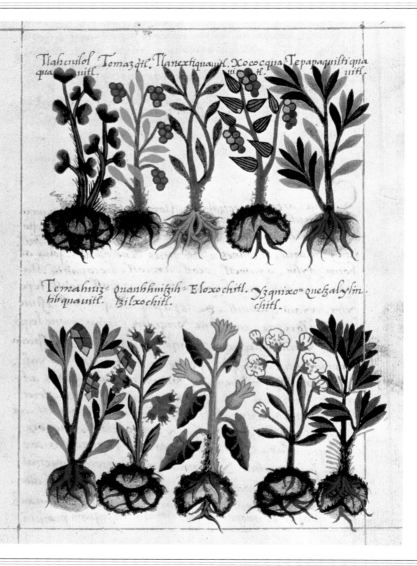

Tlahcuilol Tomazqtl. Tlanextiquauitl. Xococqua Tepapaquiltiqua
quauitl. iii tl. iiitl.

Temahuiz= quauhhuitzih= Eloxochitl= Yzquixo= quetzalysin
tliquauitl. Zilxochitl. chitl.

anthropologists who have studied the use of plants for healing by native populations. This knowledge often proves the source of discovery for new medicine. The rest of the work involved in developing a new medicine usually takes a considerable amount of time, time to dissect, isolate, reproduce, test and just occasionally to find something of value. The latest discovery in modern herbalism lies in the field of plant hormones. Certain plants contain molecules that are less aggressive towards the body and more easily metabolised than synthetic hormones (created in laboratories) thus avoiding the risks usually associated with synthetic hormones.

Essential oils and their strong antibiotic properties are one of the great successes of the plant world. These are extremely powerful concentrates of active plant ingredients. Depending on the plant they come from, they have varying qualities, either analgesic, anti-fever or anti-inflammatory, but above all they are powerfully antibiotic and could represent a very interesting modern alternative to traditional antibiotics. A study published in 1995 showed that tea-tree oil has an impact on methicillin-resistant *Staphylococcus aureus* (MRSA), a bacterium that is very much on the increase in hospitals.

THE AMAZING CREATIVITY OF NATURE

Certain plants contain more than 10,000 different molecules and it has taken more than four-and-a-half billion years for the Earth to produce such richness and diversity. Every part of a plant is like a machine producing biologically-active molecules and even the most insignificant blade of grass could hide healing properties capable of being transformed into an important discovery in the laboratory. It is this potential that encourages the giants of the pharmaceutical industry to seek exclusive rights in certain regions of the world, sometimes with government support.

MEDICINAL PLANTS
The Mexican medicinal plant, tepezcohuite, was discovered by Western chemists quite recently, when it was used to treat victims of the earthquake which destroyed much of Mexico city in 1985.

During the earthquake in Mexico in 1985, many thousands of injured people were kept waiting for medical help. They were treated with *tepezcohuitean*, an old remedy well-known to the Aztecs. This is the bark of a small variety of mimosa that the Aztecs called the 'skin tree'. In powder form it helps to heal wounds at a surprising rate. Soon after the earthquake, the world of science turned its focus upon tepezcohuite and discovered that it possessed an astonishing biological richness responsible for stimulating the growth of skin cells and halting the process of degeneration. Mexican tepezcohuite plantations are now under armed guard, to protect what has become an important national resource.

MEDICINES OF TOMORROW

Periwinkle, yew, digitalis, echinacea and ginkgo biloba are among the most modern treatments available for some of the major diseases in today's world, such as cancer, AIDS, degenerative illnesses and cardio-vascular diseases. There is always the possibility of making new discoveries as long as the plant world continues to thrive. Fortunately, there are still areas that are virtually untouched, where unique ecosystems have been preserved. This is the case in the Amazonian *Tepuis*. These sacred mountains were only discovered fairly recently, some of them less than 50 years ago. Since then, 9,400 plant species have been identified, of which 40 per cent are unknown elsewhere in the world.

The discovery of new plants is just the very beginning of the work. It takes five to ten years of research to find a truly innovative medicine and then two years of testing on animals. After that, there is, on average, another two years of testing on volunteers, followed by four years of clinical studies on patients. Finally, providing the medicine has proved to be effective and possesses no unwelcome side effects, authorisation must be given by the government before the product can be put on the market.

In certain cases, there is little in common between the original plant and the final medicine. In fact, phytochemistry, the chemistry of plants, allows the molecular components to be isolated from the plant extract and to be transformed in structure so that they are suited to a specific use. This is known as hemisynthesis. Whether they are half-plant or half-chemical, these hybrid medicines owe their existence to the plant world which inspired their creation. The work of biochemists goes hand in hand with that of botanists and agricultural engineers. When a medicine that has originated from a plant is launched on the market, the role of the laboratories is not over as a steady supply of good quality prime ingredients is still needed. Thousands of tons of fresh plants pass through laboratories every year. These may be either mixed with solvents, heated, or subjected to evaporation and may arrive on the chemist's shelves as whole plants, extracts, homeopathic dilutions, subtle extracts, hemisynthetic medicines or phytochemical products.

Despite all the scientific research that is being carried out on plants, they have still not yet yielded all their secrets. It is this fact that gives us hope that one day scientists may be able to offer us a future free from illness.

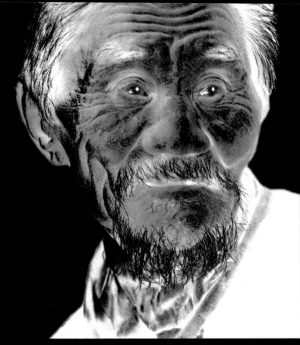

LOOK

SHAMANISM IS A FORM OF ETHNIC RELIGION BASED ON THE BELIEF IN GOOD AND EVIL SPIRITS WHICH IS STILL VERY MUCH ALIVE TODAY, NOTABLY IN SIBERIA. TINGED WITH MAGIC, THE SHAMAN CALLS UPON THE SPIRIT OF PLANTS TO HELP HEAL THE SICK.

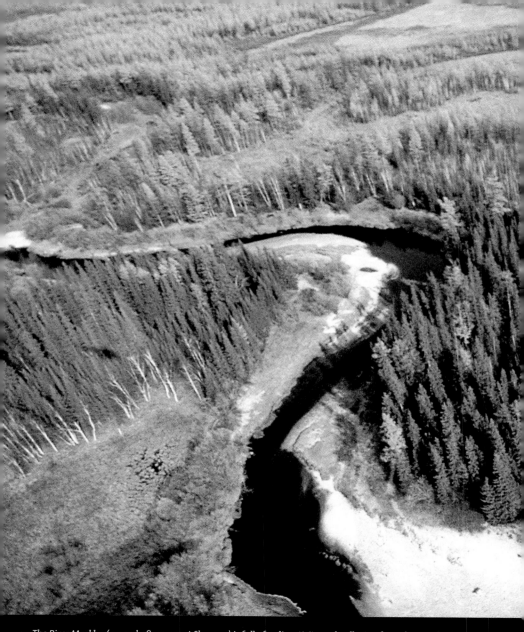

The River Markha (named after a great Shaman) is full of radioactivity and pollution from diamond mines

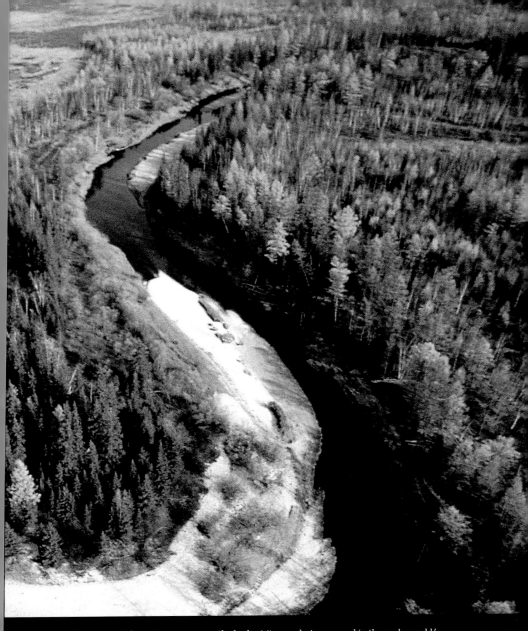

'When you lean out over the water you can see the bad spirits wandering around in the underworld.'

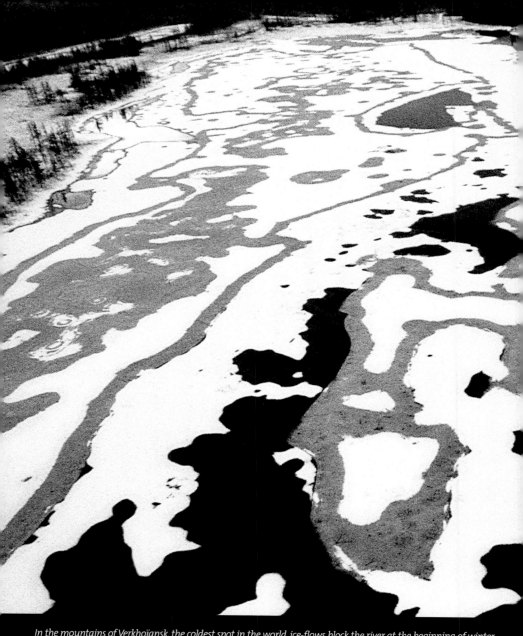

In the mountains of Verkhoïansk, the coldest spot in the world, ice-flows block the river at the beginning of winter.

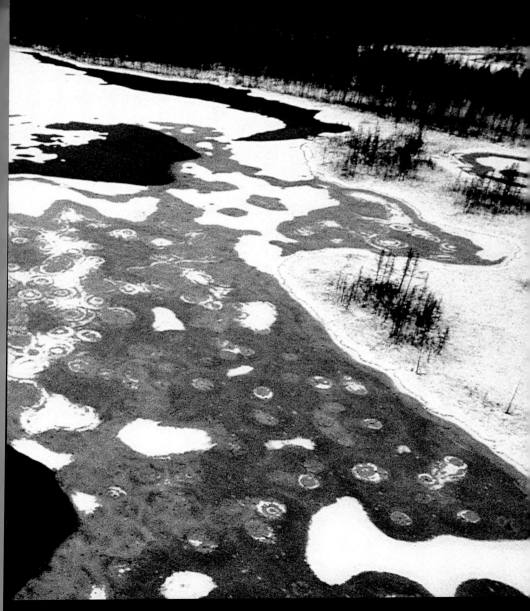

The Shamans say, 'spirits are everywhere; if you know how to look, you will see them.'

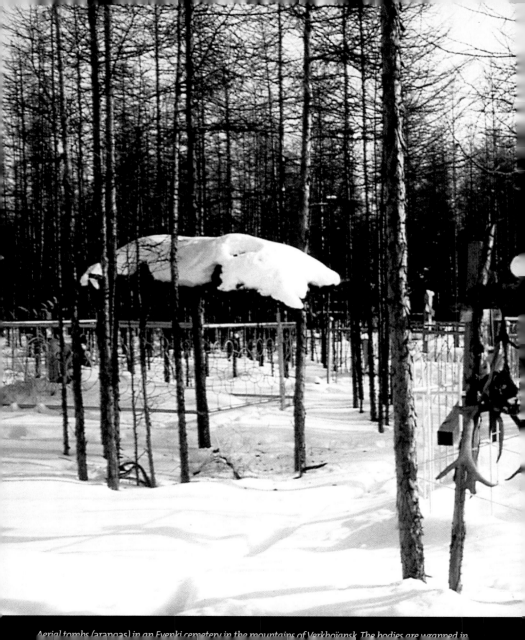

Aerial tombs (arangas) in an Evenki cemetery in the mountains of Verkhoïansk. The bodies are wrapped in

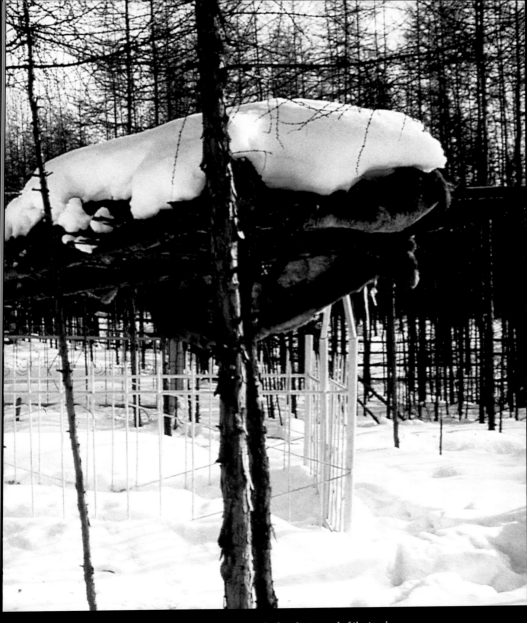

reindeer hide. The antlers of a sacrificed reindeer are attached to the top end of the tomb.

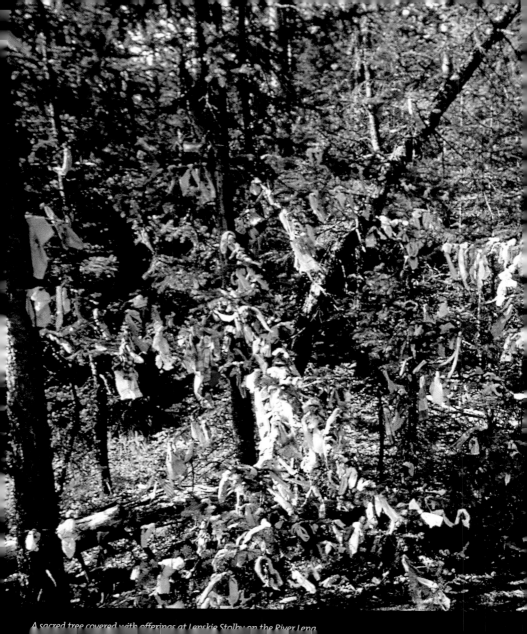

A sacred tree covered with offerings at Lenskie Stolby on the River Lena.

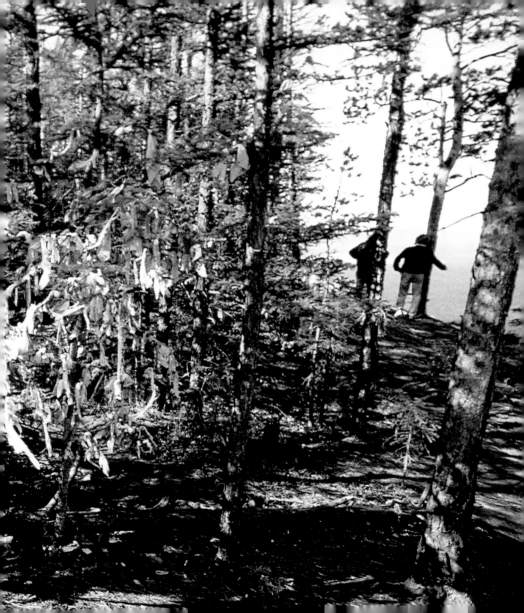

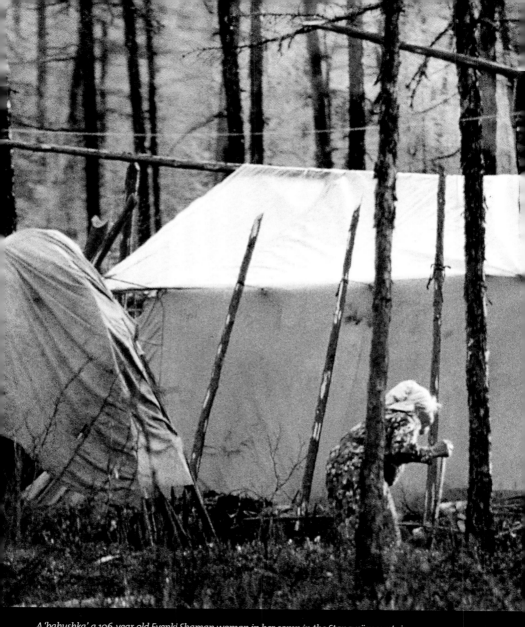

A 'babushka' a 106-year-old Evenki Shaman woman in her camp in the Stanovoï mountains.

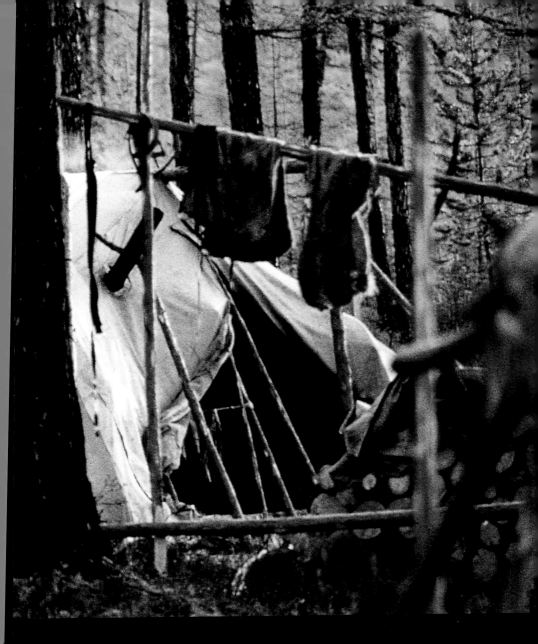

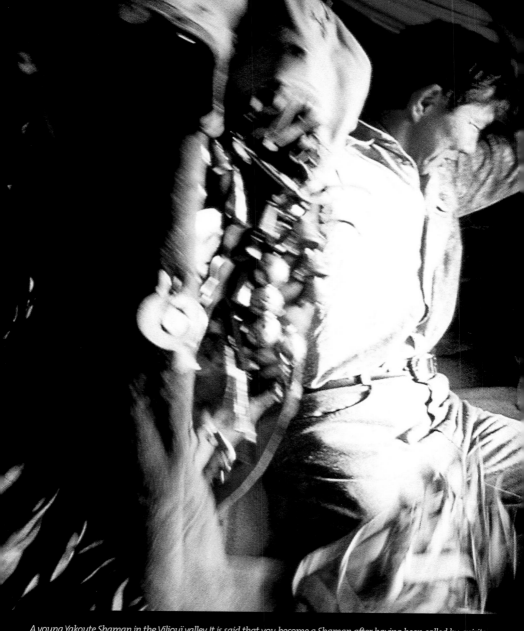

A young Yakoute Shaman in the Viliouï valley. It is said that you become a Shaman after having been called by spirits

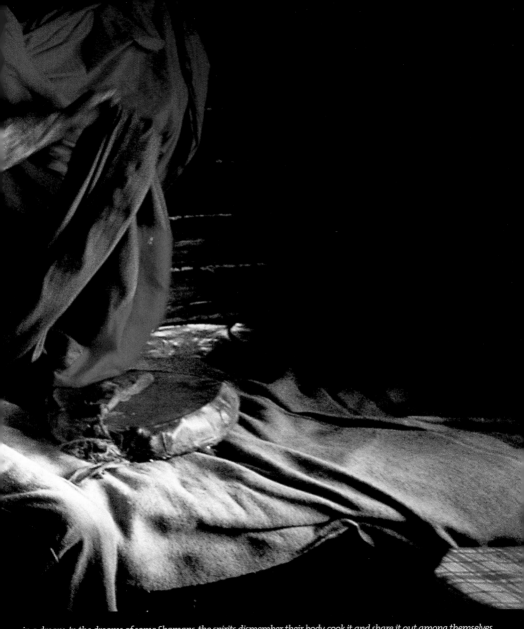

in a dream. In the dreams of some Shamans, the spirits dismember their body, cook it and share it out among themselves.

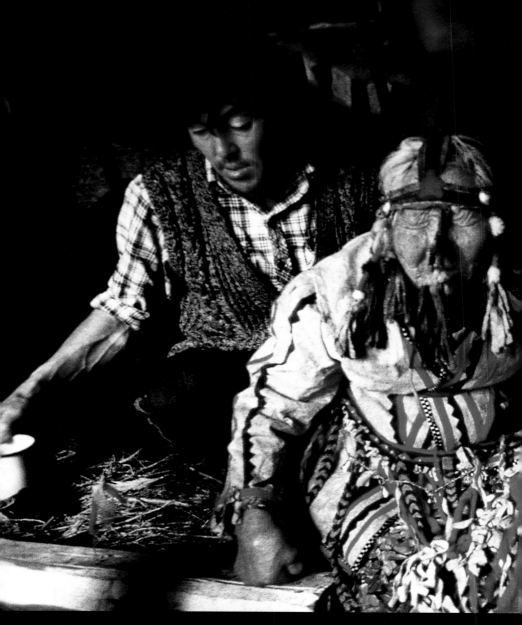

A 'babushka' during an important seance (kamlanië), with her great-grandson Egor on the drum and Volodia,

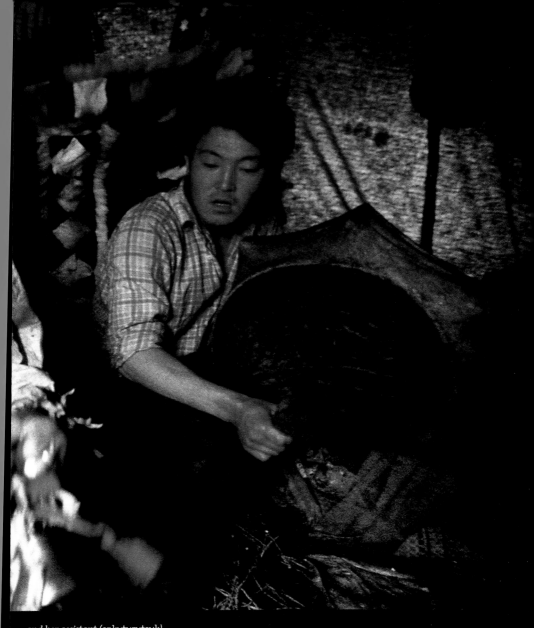

and her assistant (or kuturutsuk).

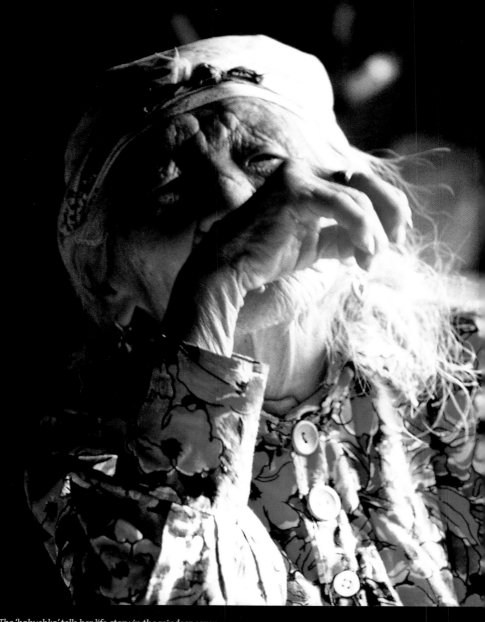

The 'babushka' tells her life-story in the reindeer camp.

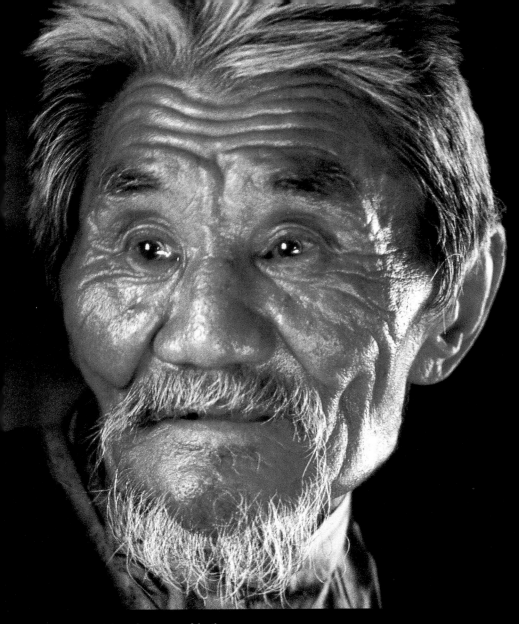

Matveï Afanasiev, a Yakoute hunter, son of the Shaman.

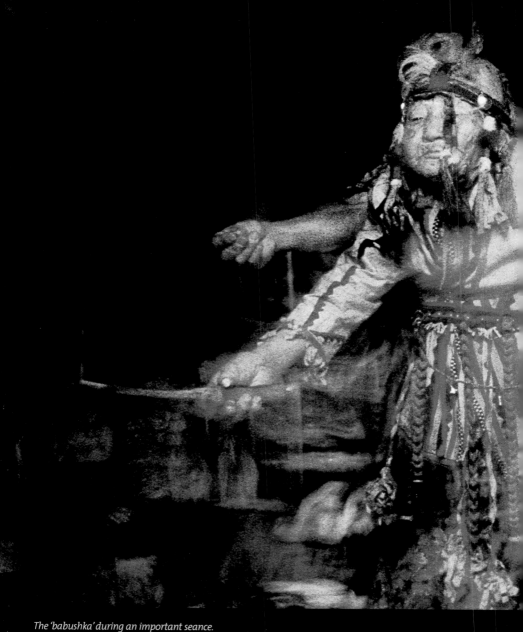

The 'babushka' during an important seance.

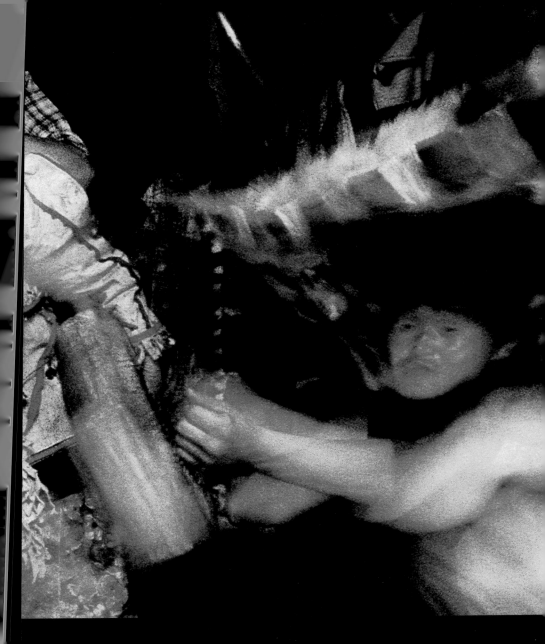

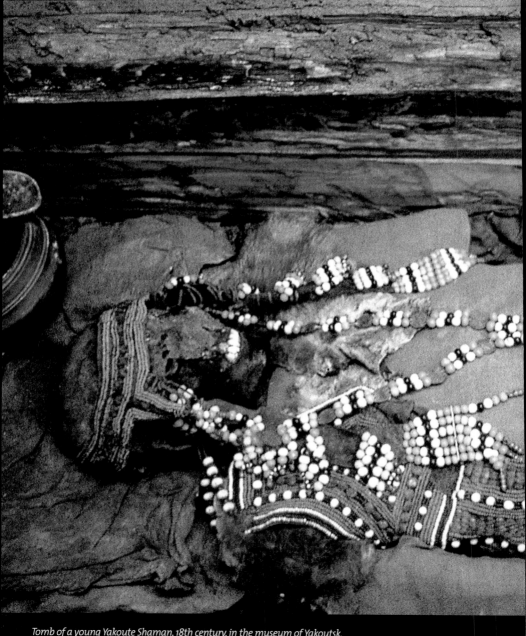

Tomb of a young Yakoute Shaman, 18th century, in the museum of Yakoutsk.

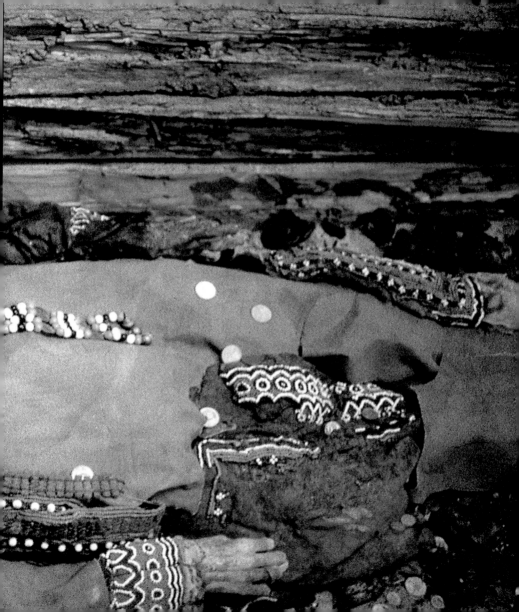

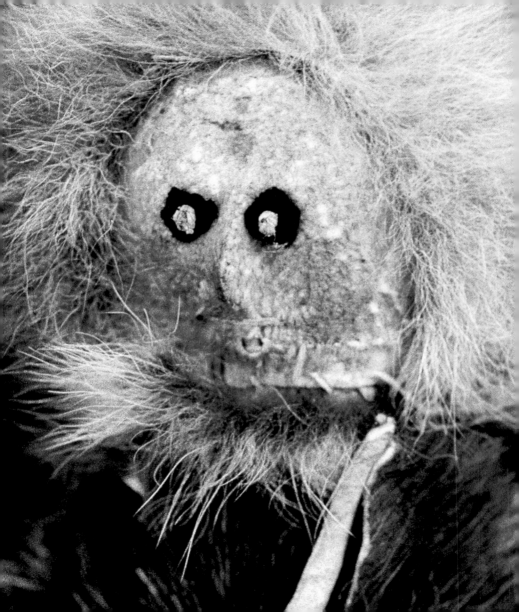

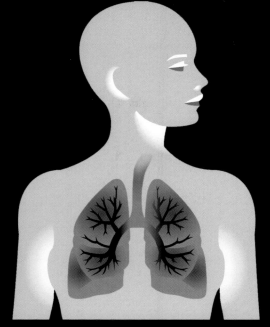

IN PRACTICE

WHAT ARE DECOCTIONS? HOW DO YOU USE INFUSIONS AND ESSENTIAL OILS?
WHAT IS AROMATHERAPY? HOW DO PLANTS AFFECT OUR BODIES?
THE MOST COMMONLY USED PLANTS IN HERBAL MEDICINE
AND HOW THEY CAN BE USED TO HEAL.

The whole plant

There is goodness in every part of a plant. Nothing should be thrown away. Medicinal plants can contain active therapeutic ingredients in every single part: leaves, flowers, buds, stalks, bark and roots. But certain rules have to be followed, especially when harvesting and storing.

Storage

Any fermentation partly destroys the active ingredients. This is why, once picked, the plant should be dried rapidly. Air drying is preferable. Alternatively, very fleshy or woody parts can be dried in an oven.

Dried plants can be kept for about a year, preferably in glass bottles that give protection from germs.

HARVEST TIME

1. Whether harvesting the root, bulb, tuber, or even a rhizome, the best time to do so is during the autumn, when the roots have taken up everything they need from the earth to get through the winter. It's also possible to harvest in early spring, before the plants have used up their energy in producing leaves and flowers.

2. Whatever the plant, the leaves should be harvested when they are fully out, but just before the flower buds appear, as these use up a major part of the active ingredients in growing.

3. Buds should be harvested as soon as they appear, before the sap mounts.

4. Flowers or flower-heads (bunches of small flowers at the top of the plant) should be harvested as soon as the buds come into flower, as this is when flowers have the highest concentration of active ingredients.

5. Fruits and berries should be picked as soon as they are ripe; they lose their active ingredients as they get older.

6. Whatever their size, stalks are best picked in winter when the sap is dormant.

7. Sapwood is the youngest part of the trunks and branches of trees and bushes. It is situated just beneath the bark where the last layers of wood are still fresh and living. Sapwood should be collected in winter when the sap is dormant.

8. For the same reason, bark, like stalks, should be collected in winter before the plant becomes active again.

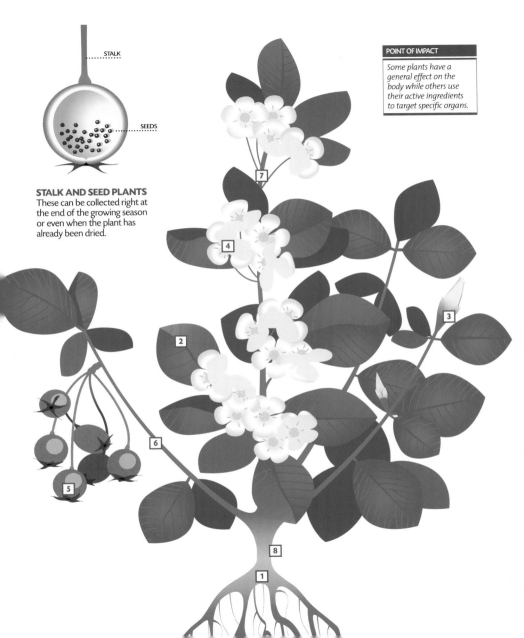

STALK

SEEDS

STALK AND SEED PLANTS
These can be collected right at
the end of the growing season
or even when the plant has
already been dried.

POINT OF IMPACT

*Some plants have a
general effect on the
body while others use
their active ingredients
to target specific organs.*

Traditional uses

Some plants dissolve active ingredients readily in water, whereas the active ingredients of others are more difficult to obtain.

Preparations

Preparing a herbal tea may be enough to release the active ingredients but there are quite a few plants that need to be boiled for up to 20 minutes. Macerating plants in wine allows alcohol-soluble ingredients to be collected, but some recalcitrant plants will only release their precious ingredients in stronger alcoholic preparations. In this case, more complex procedures are needed which are difficult to carry out at home.

Dried plants

Whatever preparation you are making, it should always be made with dried plants. This is because the active ingredients are locked in the plant cells, which are like little boxes made of cellulose. When the plant is fresh, the heat of the water is not sufficient to break down the cellulose walls and some of the active ingredients stay enclosed within the plant. However, when the plant is dry, the walls of the little boxes are already cracked and it is easy for the active ingredients to diffuse in the water or in the solvent.

Herbal teas (tisanes)

Boil some water and pour it on to the plants while it is still boiling. Then stir and cover. Depending on the plant, the time of infusion varies from five and 20 minutes. Filter with a fine sieve.

Decoctions

Put the plants in cold (but not icy) water and leave to settle for a few minutes. Bring to the boil and boil for one to 20 minutes depending on the plant. Filter with a fine sieve.

Macerations

Soak the plants in a container of mineral water at room temperature and away from direct sunlight. Leave for between two and ten days according to the plant, stirring carefully every day. Strain and press to extract all the liquid.

Tinctures

Macerate the plant in good quality wine in a cool, dark place for two to three weeks depending on the plant. Strain and press to extract all the liquid.

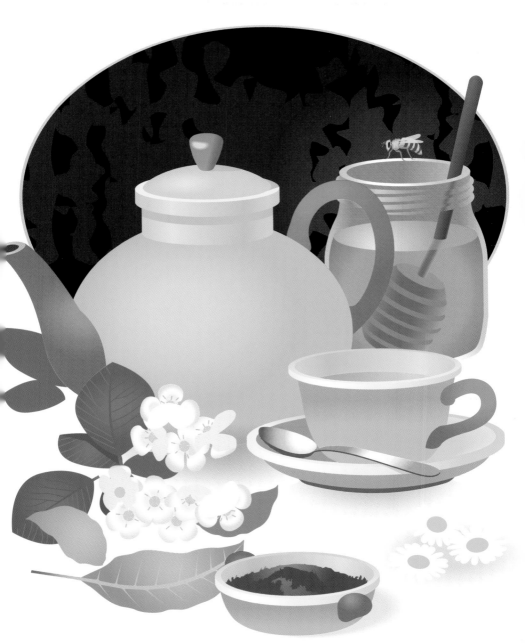

The beneficial effects of tea

Black or green?

Whatever the colour of the tea, the plant from which it comes is the same, *Camellia sinensi*: the difference between black and green teas lies in the method of harvesting. The best tea (Pekoe) is harvested when the bud is just beginning to lengthen into the shape of a small cigar. If it is harvested later or when the bud has a large bouquet of leaves the quality is inferior.

Green tea

This is very rich in tannins, especially catechin which slows down the build-up of cholesterol and also acts as an antidiuretic. Studies on mice have shown that daily consumption of green tea halts the growth of 87 per cent of skin cancers, 58 per cent of stomach cancers and 56 per cent of lung cancers. This antitumour action is due to a high concentration of polyphenols (antioxidants which prevent cell degeneration) and of epigallocatechin gallate (ten times higher than in black tea), a substance that slows down one of the enzymes responsible for the growth of tumours. (Professor Conney, University of New Jersey; Professor Fujiki, Japan National Cancer Research Institute).

Tea is the most popular beverage derived from a plant in the world and is the number-one breakfast drink. It is so popular that it is easy to forget its therapeutic qualities. However, tea is a truly medicinal plant and science has recently discovered some more of its therapeutic properties.

Exotic origins

According to legend, in 2737 BC, the Chinese Emperor Chin Nong, the father of Chinese medicine, was getting ready to drink his daily bowl of hot water when a few leaves from the tea bush under which he was resting fell into his cup. The rest is history and a cup of tea has become a symbol of conviviality and hospitality everywhere; witness our own British tea time, Indian *'tcha'* Arabian mint tea and the Japanese tea ceremony, to name but a few.

The virtues of tea

Tea is a stimulating, diuretic, digestive, purgative, anticholesterol, slimming and even in some cases an anticancerous drink. It contains vitamins, trace elements, fluoride, an anticaries and an antidecalcification substance as well as theine, caffeine, and theophylline and theobromine which are both stimulating and diuretic substances.

Black tea

This contains many flavonoids, artery protectors that reduce the risk of cardio-vascular disease. Its high concentration of vitamin B9 (folic acid) strengthens the vessel walls. (According to a Dutch study carried out over 15 years on 552 people.)

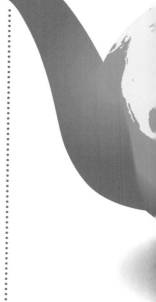

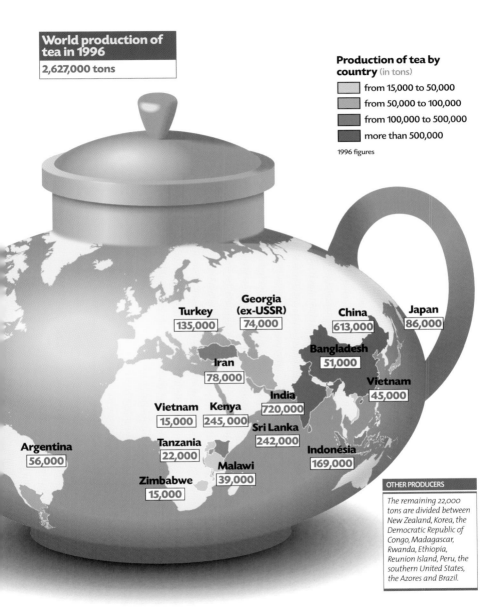

World production of tea in 1996
2,627,000 tons

Production of tea by country (in tons)

- from 15,000 to 50,000
- from 50,000 to 100,000
- from 100,000 to 500,000
- more than 500,000

1996 figures

Turkey 135,000
Georgia (ex-USSR) 74,000
China 613,000
Japan 86,000
Bangladesh 51,000
Iran 78,000
Vietnam 45,000
India 720,000
Vietnam 15,000
Kenya 245,000
Sri Lanka 242,000
Argentina 56,000
Tanzania 22,000
Indonésia 169,000
Malawi 39,000
Zimbabwe 15,000

OTHER PRODUCERS

The remaining 22,000 tons are divided between New Zealand, Korea, the Democratic Republic of Congo, Madagascar, Rwanda, Ethiopia, Reunion Island, Peru, the southern United States, the Azores and Brazil.

Modern methods of presentation

Today, plants are sold in many different forms. To make an informed choice you need to know what the different products contain.

Which preparation?

Some treatments favour the extraction of alcohol-soluble active ingredients, and are best suited to those plants that contain them in high quantities, while others are water-soluble. Very fragile active ingredients are better preserved by freezing. The choice of drops, capsules or ampoules depends on the individual.

Irradiated plants

Some laboratories irradiate dried plants to prevent micro-organisms from developing. They are treated with gamma-rays: an effective method as far as hygiene is concerned but what is not known yet is if this treatment destroys certain active ingredients.

Tinctures

The plant is macerated in a mixture of alcohol and water. In this way, the active ingredients pass into the liquid whether they are soluble in water or in alcohol. The resulting substance is dried and strained.

The plant extract is adjusted so that the active ingredient is always the same, no matter which plant is used, its origin or the time of harvest. Finally the extract is dried, reduced to a powder and put into capsules.

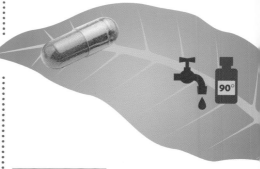

Powders

Plants are dried, then crushed and sieved to get rid of impurities. Commonly supplied in capsules.

Essential substances from fresh plants

The plants are crushed and frozen. Then the mixture is stabilised in alcohol vapour to preserve all the active ingredients, even those which have been damaged by the drying process. The liquid is cooled and bottled.

Distillation

Plants are macerated in a mixture of water and alcohol, heated and put into a centrifuge to isolate the active substances, which are then collected and bottled.

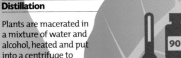

Freezing and crushing

Plants are frozen rapidly to a very low temperature; then reduced to a powder. This avoids using heat which affects certain fragile active ingredients. The powder is then put into capsules.

Alcohol-based extractions

Plants are macerated in alcohol to extract the alcohol-soluble substances. The time of maceration varies according to the plant; it could last up to three weeks. The mixture is then strained and the resulting strained liquid preserved.

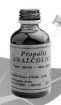

Antistress plants

Stress is now enemy number one in modern life. Seven out of ten people admit to being stressed. Broadly speaking, the symptoms are anxiety, agitation and sleeplessness.

Conquer stress

To combat stress we take medicines that affect the brain, mind-changing drugs such as tranquillisers, and sleeping tablets. Unfortunately, there is a danger of addiction. Gradually the body gets used to them, they become less effective and consequently the dose has to be increased. After a few months it is impossible to do without them. To avoid becoming dependent on these drugs, there is another option – antistress plants.

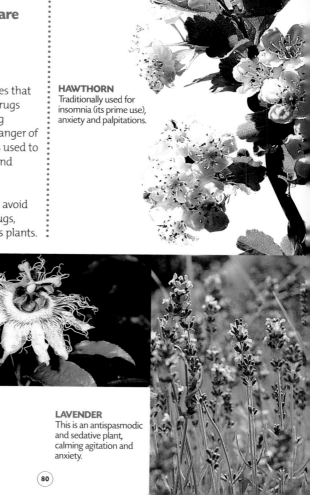

HAWTHORN
Traditionally used for insomnia (its prime use), anxiety and palpitations.

THE PASSION FLOWER
This is a powerful antistress plant that calms the overworked and helps them to sleep peacefully. However, care must be taken not to drink too much as it can cause migraine. Stop the treatment or reduce the dose at the first sign of any migraine symptoms.

LAVENDER
This is an antispasmodic and sedative plant, calming agitation and anxiety.

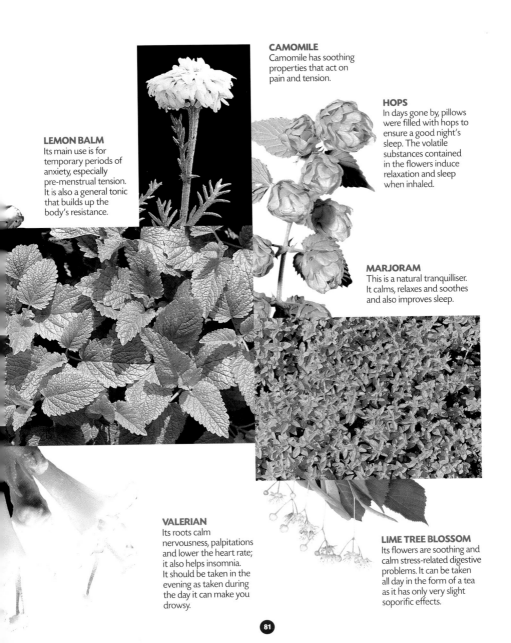

CAMOMILE
Camomile has soothing properties that act on pain and tension.

HOPS
In days gone by, pillows were filled with hops to ensure a good night's sleep. The volatile substances contained in the flowers induce relaxation and sleep when inhaled.

LEMON BALM
Its main use is for temporary periods of anxiety, especially pre-menstrual tension. It is also a general tonic that builds up the body's resistance.

MARJORAM
This is a natural tranquilliser. It calms, relaxes and soothes and also improves sleep.

VALERIAN
Its roots calm nervousness, palpitations and lower the heart rate; it also helps insomnia. It should be taken in the evening as taken during the day it can make you drowsy.

LIME TREE BLOSSOM
Its flowers are soothing and calm stress-related digestive problems. It can be taken all day in the form of a tea as it has only very slight soporific effects.

St John's wort:
a plant to combat depression

St John's wort is effective as an antidepressant. It has none of the dependency problems or secondary effects associated with traditional antidepressant drugs.

A natural antidepressant

In days gone by, people who were said to be possessed by spirits were made to inhale vapours from St John's wort in order to expel their demons. Today, we know for certain that this plant aids sufferers from depression. Various studies have confirmed that its effects are at least equal to those of chemical antidepressants, with far fewer secondary effects and dependency problems.

Extraction by alcohol

The flower-heads are macerated in alcohol and then the liquid is evaporated. The extracts contain large quantities of hypericine, the ingredient responsible for the antidepressive action. The preparation that is to go into the capsules is tested and adjusted so that the capsules always contain the same percentage of hypericine. The usual daily dose prescribed is between 300 and 900 mg (0.01 and 0.03 ounces) of extract according to the gravity of the depression.

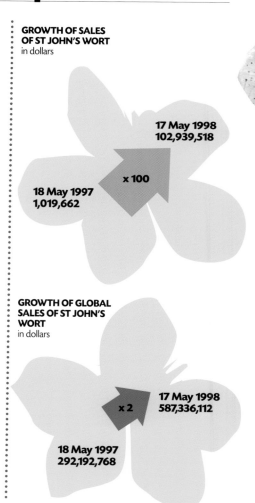

**GROWTH OF SALES
OF ST JOHN'S WORT**
in dollars

17 May 1998
102,939,518

x 100

18 May 1997
1,019,662

**GROWTH OF GLOBAL
SALES OF ST JOHN'S
WORT**
in dollars

17 May 1998
587,336,112

x 2

18 May 1997
292,192,768

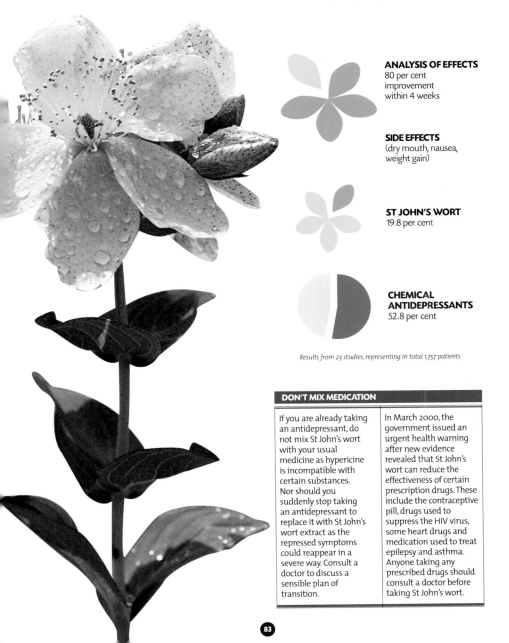

ANALYSIS OF EFFECTS
80 per cent
improvement
within 4 weeks

SIDE EFFECTS
(dry mouth, nausea,
weight gain)

ST JOHN'S WORT
19.8 per cent

CHEMICAL
ANTIDEPRESSANTS
52.8 per cent

Results from 23 studies, representing in total 1,757 patients

DON'T MIX MEDICATION

If you are already taking an antidepressant, do not mix St John's wort with your usual medicine as hypericine is incompatible with certain substances. Nor should you suddenly stop taking an antidepressant to replace it with St John's wort extract as the repressed symptoms could reappear in a severe way. Consult a doctor to discuss a sensible plan of transition.

In March 2000, the government issued an urgent health warning after new evidence revealed that St John's wort can reduce the effectiveness of certain prescription drugs. These include the contraceptive pill, drugs used to suppress the HIV virus, some heart drugs and medication used to treat epilepsy and asthma. Anyone taking any prescribed drugs should consult a doctor before taking St John's wort.

With the blessing of science

Over the past 20 years plants have been the subject of extensive scientific studies which have both confirmed their efficacy and led to the discovery of new applications. Here are a few stars of current research.

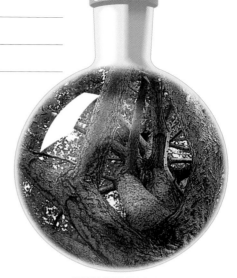

The Pacific yew

Between 1950 and 1980, the American National Cancer Institute conducted an extensive programme of study on the effects of 35,000 plants on cancer. It was within this framework that in 1967, scientists discovered the antitumour properties of the Pacific yew.

The active substance, paclitaxel, is concentrated in the bark and the needles of the tree. The effectiveness of this substance, taxol, on certain cancers such as breast, bronchial and brain cancer has been proven. It is estimated that 30 per cent of ovarian cancers resistant to traditional treatments can be cured in this way.

THE PACIFIC YEW TREE

Ginkgo biloba

A plant that has outlived the dinosaurs. It has been in existence in an identical form for more than 200 million years having survived all the Earth's climatic changes and catastrophes, including the atomic bomb at Hiroshima. Research has revealed its richness in flavonoids and terpenes. Among the latter category are ginkgolides that have

antiageing properties. They trap free radicals that are responsible for the wearing out of cells and improve blood circulation, especially to the brain.

Today, the only problem for the laboratories is that the active ingredients are very difficult to reproduce artificially. They are thus obliged, for the moment, to continue to produce medicines from natural plant extracts.

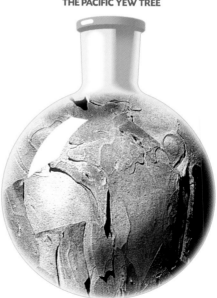

GINKGO BILOBA

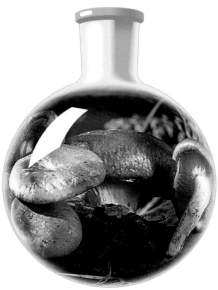

SHIITAKE

Shiitake

This edible mushroom has been included in the oriental pharmacopoeia for several centuries. Recent research, like that of Professor Yamamura (University of California) has shown that it is rich in lentinan, a rare substance that has strong immune system stimulating and antiviral properties. Shiitake is an excellent remedy for tired immune systems. It can also be used to protect against germs and viruses.

Other research, like that of Doctor Abrams (Centre of Research San Francisco UC) has shown that shiitake allows the regeneration of immune cells in AIDS patients. Of course, it cannot alone constitute a cure against this disease but it is an effective complementary treatment.

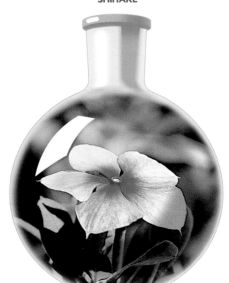

MADAGASCAN PERIWINKLE

Madagascan periwinkle

This tropical shrub, which is scarcely 50 cm (15 in) high, is used by local healers as an antidiabetic. Recent studies have shown that one of its 60 alkaloids, vincamine, slows down cell multiplication in certain types of cancer.

A medicine, Navelbine, has been developed from this plant substance. Clinical studies have shown that it is effective in 60 per cent of breast cancers resistant to traditional chemotherapy. Today it is officially used in about 50 countries, including the United States.

The lungs of the planet

It is thought that there are millions of species of plant yet to be discovered, mainly in the rich tropical forests that remain little explored. These species contain substances that may give rise to the medicines of tomorrow. Unfortunately, the flora of the world is in danger, threatened by deforestation, pollution and global warming.

Concern for the future

In spite of recent international agreements and cries of alarm from scientists and ecologists, tropical and equatorial forests are disappearing at the rate of 5,000 sq m (60 sq yds) per second. During the last 200,000 years, the natural rhythm of extinction was just one species every two years whereas now a species disappears from the planet every 15 minutes. Meanwhile, the health of future generations is going up in smoke.

Plants are vital

Three out of four medicines come from plants, either directly (made from plant extracts) or indirectly (reproduced chemically from plant molecules). Thus we have all, at one time or another, benefited from the healing power of plants, though we might not be aware of it.

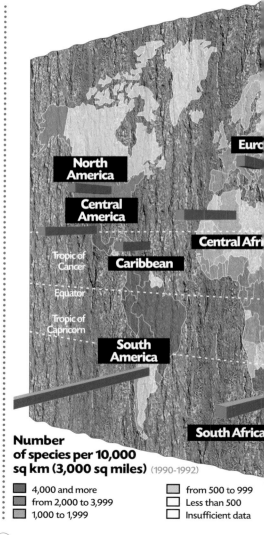

Number of species per 10,000 sq km (3,000 sq miles) (1990-1992)

- 4,000 and more
- from 2,000 to 3,999
- 1,000 to 1,999
- from 500 to 999
- Less than 500
- Insufficient data

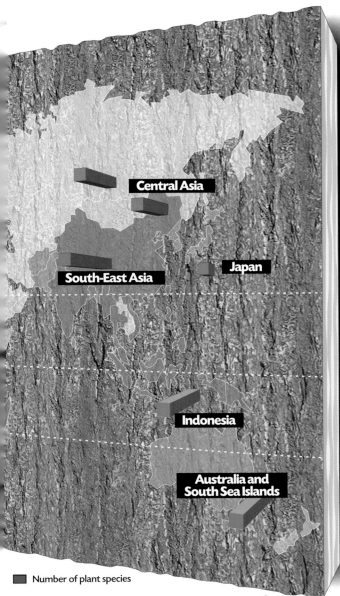

Central Asia

South-East Asia

Japan

Indonesia

Australia and
South Sea Islands

Number of plant species

Global warming

Since the last ice age (13,000 years ago) the temperature at the Earth's surface has increased by 4°C (39°F). This increase was enough to change the climate of Europe from a polar one to a temperate one. However, since the 19th century it has taken a mere 130 years of industrial activity in the West to cause an increase in temperature of another 0.5°C (33°F) degrees.

Threatened forests

Parks and nature reserves account for only 1.6 per cent of the total surface area of forests in the world. An astonishing 8,750 species of tropical trees are currently threatened with extinction. Since 1980, the forests of the world have diminished by nearly 50 million hectares (1,235 million acres). Between 1990 and 1995, 3,750,000 hectares (9,262,500 acres) of forest disappeared in Africa, 4,200,000 hectares (10,374,000 acres) in Asia and 5,800,000 hectares (14,326,000 acres) in Latin America.

More statistics

Of the enormous number of plants that have been recorded as being used for medicinal purposes, 4,500 grow in Europe, 6,500 in South-East Asia, 1,300 in the Amazon, 5,000 in China and 2,500 in India.

Essential oils: plant concentrates

These extracts of aromatic plants are very powerful. The active ingredients are up to 100 times more concentrated in an essential oil than in a fresh plant.

The action of essential oils

Their effects are different to those of the plants themselves. Valerian is used in herbalism for its calming properties, but the essence of valerian does not have these qualities. The sedative substances, valtrates, are too heavy to be carried by vapour during distillation. Similarly, garlic essence contains a substance that is not present in fresh garlic. This substance slows down the accumulation of platelets in the blood and is produced during distillation by the effects of heat and moisture.

Properties of oils

Depending on which plant the oil comes from, an oil can be described as being anti-inflammatory, antiseptic, antiviral, antibiotic, diuretic, analgesic, antifungal or antirheumatic. It can also act as an aid to healing wounds, as a stimulant, a digestive, an expectorant and a laxative. It can help to heal the liver, reduce a high temperature, to soothe and to constrict or dilate blood vessels.

HOW TO CHOOSE ESSENTIAL OILS

- Read the label carefully
- Check the origin of the oil
- Avoid synthetic or semi-synthetic oils. These are chemical copies of active ingredients or chemical copies mixed with natural oils. They will not have the therapeutic properties of natural essences and can cause reactions such as itching or nausea.

- Choose 100 per cent natural oils (mixtures of essences) or 100 per cent pure and natural (single essences).
- Organic oils, which are 100 per cent pure and natural, come from plants that have been cultivated according to the rules of organic farming, ie without pesticides or chemical fertiliser.

Stalks, branches and roots

The hardest and woodiest parts of the plants are macerated in a solvent, usually alcohol. After a period of time (the length depends on the plant), the solvent, along with the now diffused components, is collected and then strained. This is called solvent extraction.

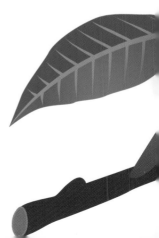

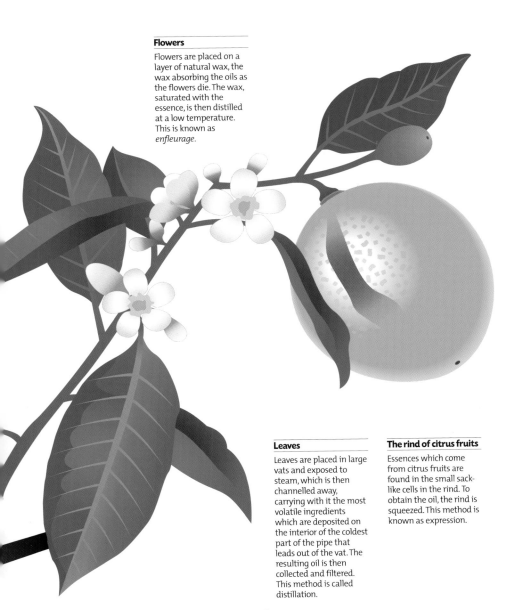

Flowers

Flowers are placed on a layer of natural wax, the wax absorbing the oils as the flowers die. The wax, saturated with the essence, is then distilled at a low temperature. This is known as *enfleurage*.

Leaves

Leaves are placed in large vats and exposed to steam, which is then channelled away, carrying with it the most volatile ingredients which are deposited on the interior of the coldest part of the pipe that leads out of the vat. The resulting oil is then collected and filtered. This method is called distillation.

The rind of citrus fruits

Essences which come from citrus fruits are found in the small sack-like cells in the rind. To obtain the oil, the rind is squeezed. This method is known as expression.

How to use essential oils

Essential oils can find their way into the body by means of oral consumption, inhalation or through the skin. They can be used in a variety of ways, depending on the manner in which they enter the body. In all cases, active ingredients are distributed by the blood to those cells needing them.

To freshen and scent the air

You might want to buy an oil diffuser. This is a small electrical appliance that releases essential oils slowly into the atmosphere. The scent is gently absorbed by the body. This method is ideal for perfuming a living space, either by introducing soothing scents in the evening or stimulating ones in the morning.

Massage

Adding a few drops of essential oil to massage oil makes this a more therapeutic practice. The active ingredients pass through the skin and circulate in the blood stream by means of the numerous small blood vessels which supply the skin.

Oral consumption

Taking oils by mouth is an effective method but can be dangerous if the essential oils are toxic. The dosage is prescribed in drops and should be strictly adhered to. If you are treating yourself do not take essential oils in this way: it should only be used if medically prescribed. There are some oils that are available in capsules which are easier to administer, but they still need to be taken with care. The active ingredients enter the body through the digestive system and pass into the blood stream through the intestinal wall.

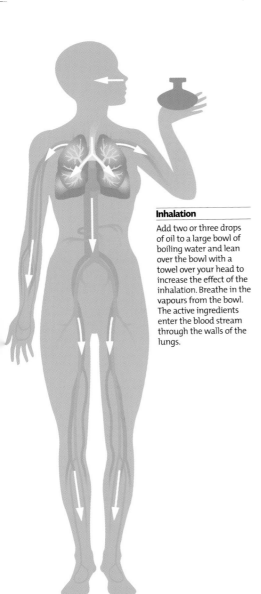

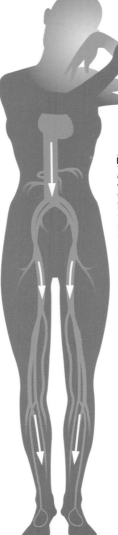

Inhalation

Add two or three drops of oil to a large bowl of boiling water and lean over the bowl with a towel over your head to increase the effect of the inhalation. Breathe in the vapours from the bowl. The active ingredients enter the blood stream through the walls of the lungs.

Bathing

As oils are not soluble in water, they should not be thrown straight into the bath. They'll just float rather than mix with the water and could irritate the skin. Mix the oil (ten drops) with a little milk before adding it to the bath water, preferably just under the taps to make sure it will be evenly distributed. The active ingredients will enter the body in two ways: through the skin and by inhalation, as the heat will cause the most volatile substances to evaporate into the atmosphere of the room.

Massage using essential oils

Choose stimulating oils such as aniseed, jasmine and lemon. Start by massaging the toes, one by one, then use circular motions on the ball of the foot beginning in the middle.

Finally, massage the foot all over, as far as the ankles. The ball of the foot is very rich in nerve endings which makes this type of massage particularly effective.

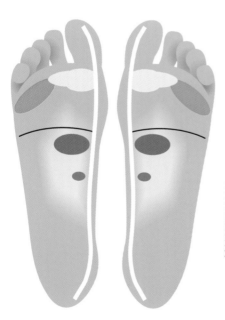

THE COLOURED AREAS REPRESENT OTHER ZONES THAT CAN BE MASSAGED WITH CIRCULAR MOVEMENTS.

Only a few drops of essential oil are needed to transform a simple relaxing massage into a really useful healing tool.

Preparing for a massage

Prepare a base mixture of oils (grape seed, almond, jojoba, corn, apricot kernel, avocado) according to taste.

For each massage, put a large tablespoon of the base oil into a bowl and add about ten drops of the essential oil of your choice. You can create a mixture of up to three essential oils, as long as they have compatible properties.

Friction massage

Friction massage is the term used when the massage is confined to precise areas. The effect is more powerful and more precise than a straightforward massage. With the same mixture of base oils, prepare a 100 ml (3.5 fl ounces) bottle to which should be added five ml (0.17 fl ounces) of essential oils chosen for their desired effect. Then begin to massage. The solar plexus, nape of the neck, temples or legs are all suitable for this kind of massage.

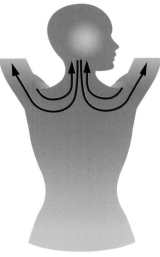

BEGIN BY MASSAGING THE BASE OF THE NAPE AND SIDES OF THE NECK WORKING FROM THE BOTTOM TO THE TOP. WORK ALONG THE SHOULDERS AND THE ARMS DOWN AS FAR AS THE ELBOWS USING SMALL CIRCULAR MOVEMENTS.

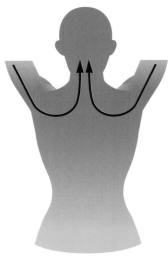

WORK UPWARDS AGAIN TO THE NECK. REPEAT FIVE TIMES.

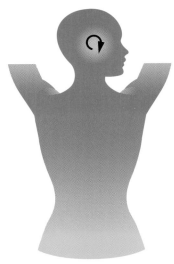

MASSAGE THE TEMPLES WITH SMALL CIRCULAR MOVEMENTS.

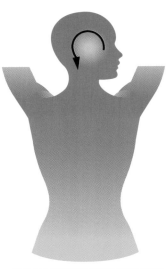

CONTINUING TO USE CIRCULAR MOVEMENTS MASSAGE DOWN AS FAR AS THE NECK.

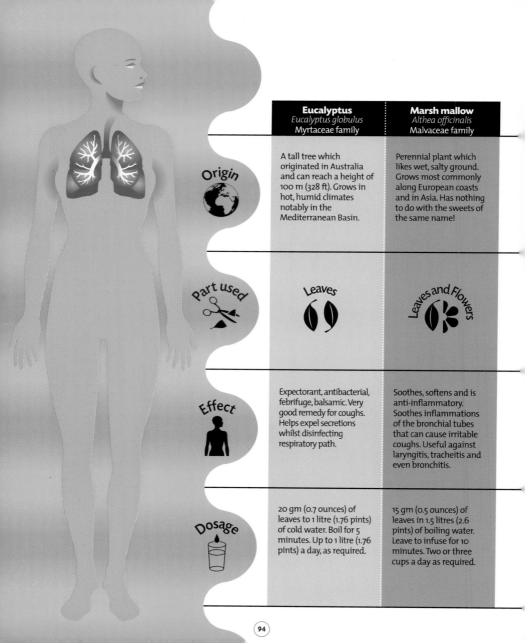

	Eucalyptus *Eucalyptus globulus* Myrtaceae family	**Marsh mallow** *Althea officinalis* Malvaceae family
Origin	A tall tree which originated in Australia and can reach a height of 100 m (328 ft). Grows in hot, humid climates notably in the Mediterranean Basin.	Perennial plant which likes wet, salty ground. Grows most commonly along European coasts and in Asia. Has nothing to do with the sweets of the same name!
Part used	Leaves	Leaves and Flowers
Effect	Expectorant, antibacterial, febrifuge, balsamic. Very good remedy for coughs. Helps expel secretions whilst disinfecting respiratory path.	Soothes, softens and is anti-inflammatory. Soothes inflammations of the bronchial tubes that can cause irritable coughs. Useful against laryngitis, tracheitis and even bronchitis.
Dosage	20 gm (0.7 ounces) of leaves to 1 litre (1.76 pints) of cold water. Boil for 5 minutes. Up to 1 litre (1.76 pints) a day, as required.	15 gm (0.5 ounces) of leaves in 1.5 litres (2.6 pints) of boiling water. Leave to infuse for 10 minutes. Two or three cups a day as required.

Plants for bronchial troubles

White Horehound *Marrubium vulgare* Labiatae family	Pine *Pinus sylvestris* Conifer family	Plantain *Plantago major* Plantaginaceae family	Meadowsweet *Filipendula ulmaria* Rosaceae family
Likes dry ground, commonly found in Europe, especially in southern regions.	Tall tree from mountainous, southern regions.	Hardy plant, found on all continents. Grows in fields and on the edge of woods.	Likes wet fields, very common in Europe.
Leaves and Flowers	Buds	Plant, roots and seeds	Whole plant
Expectorant, disinfectant, febrifuge. Disinfects the lungs, gets rid of accumulated secretions by helping to expel them. Calms dry cough attacks.	Expectorant, antiseptic, fortifying, stimulating, sudorific. Known for centuries for its efficacy against bronchial diseases. Also helps combat fatigue after infections.	Expectorant, astringent, purgative. Helps expel secretions caused by loose coughs and calms irritations caused by dry coughs.	Febrifuge, analgesic, diuretic. Contains derivatives of salicylic acid. Calms fever and relieves pain. Useful combined with other plants to treat infections of the respiratory system.
4 tablespoons to 1 litre (1.76 pints) of boiling water. Leave to infuse for 10 minutes. No more than 2 or 3 cups a day (risk of palpitations). As required.	1 tablespoon in a large bowl of cold water. Boil for 3 minutes and leave to infuse for 5 minutes. Three bowls a day, as required.	2 tablespoons in a big bowl of boiling water. Leave to infuse for 10 minutes. Two bowls a day, as required.	1 tablespoon to a big bowl of boiling water. Leave to infuse for 10 minutes. 3 half-bowls a day, between meals.

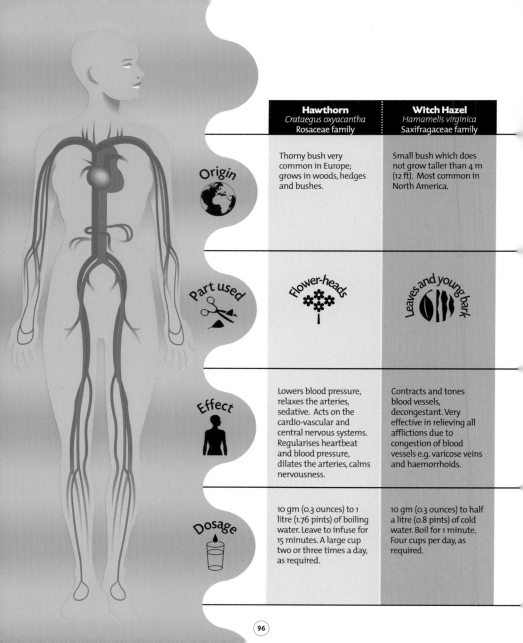

	Hawthorn *Crataegus oxyacantha* Rosaceae family	**Witch Hazel** *Hamamelis virginica* Saxifragaceae family
Origin	Thorny bush very common in Europe; grows in woods, hedges and bushes.	Small bush which does not grow taller than 4 m (12 ft). Most common in North America.
Part used	Flower-heads	Leaves and young bark
Effect	Lowers blood pressure, relaxes the arteries, sedative. Acts on the cardio-vascular and central nervous systems. Regularises heartbeat and blood pressure, dilates the arteries, calms nervousness.	Contracts and tones blood vessels, decongestant. Very effective in relieving all afflictions due to congestion of blood vessels e.g. varicose veins and haemorrhoids.
Dosage	10 gm (0.3 ounces) to 1 litre (1.76 pints) of boiling water. Leave to infuse for 15 minutes. A large cup two or three times a day, as required.	10 gm (0.3 ounces) to half a litre (0.8 pints) of cold water. Boil for 1 minute. Four cups per day, as required.

Plants which aid circulation

Horse chestnut *Aesculus hippocastanum* Hippocastanaceae family	Common melilot *Mélilotus officinalis* Leguminosae family	Olive tree *Olea europea* Oleaceae family	Vine *Vitis vinifera* Vitaceae family
Very common tree in Europe, originally from the Balkans. It can live for up to 300 years.	Small herbaceous plant common in Europe and in Asia. Prefers poor soils.	Found in the Mediterranean region. Grows in stony and poor soils and in hot dry climates.	Climbing plant, commonly found around the Mediterranean Basin and in western Asia.
Fruits Preferably picked from trees more than 3 years old.	**Flower-heads**	**Leaves**	**Leaves**
Contracts vessels, decongestant, haemostatic. Helps blood circulation and relieves varicose veins and haemorrhoids.	Anticoagulant, antiseptic, antispasmodic. Coumarin, one of its main components, has an anticoagulant effect. Prevents clots that could block arteries.	Lowers blood pressure, relaxes blood vessels, antispasmodic. Lowers heart rate and stabilises blood pressure.	Astringent, pelvic decongestant, tones blood vessels. Repairs vein walls. Helps to prevent oedema of the legs, haemorrhoids and circulatory problems connected with the menopause.
20 gm (0.6 ounces) of crushed horse chestnuts to half a litre (0.8 pints) of cold water. Boil for 5 minutes and leave to infuse for 10 minutes. Two cups a day between meals.	1 tablespoon to 1 litre (1.76 pints) of boiling water. Leave to infuse for 5 minutes. Two to three cups per day, between meals.	10 gm (0.3 ounces) per litre (1.76 pints) of cold water. Boil for 3 minutes and leave to infuse for 10 minutes. One large cup three times a day between meals.	2 tablespoons to one big bowl of boiling water. Leave to infuse for 10 minutes. Half a bowl in the morning before eating.

	Artichoke *Cynara scolymus* Composeae family	**Boldina** *Pneumus boldus* Monimiaceae family
Origin	Plant from temperate regions, known for its flower, consumed as a vegetable when it is in bud.	Small tree originating in Chile with thick, grey, ridged leaves.
Part used	Leaves	Leaves
Effect	Choleretic and diuretic. Increases the production of bile and helps its evacuation. Helpful for tired livers.	Stimulant for the liver and the digestive, choleretic and diuretic organs. Effective against liver and bladder problems.
Dosage	1 tablespoon of dried leaves to one bowl of boiling water. Leave to infuse for 10 minutes. Half a bowl before lunch and evening meal.	10 gm (0.3 ounces) per litre (1.76 pints) of boiling water. Leave to infuse for 10 minutes. One cup before lunch and evening meal.

Plants that aid digestion

Buckthorn *Rhammus frangula* Rhamnaceae family	Mallow *Malva sylvestris – rotundifolia* Malvaceae family	Peppermint *Menta piperita* Labiatae family	Rosemary *Rosmarinus officinalis* Labiatae family
Shrub commonly found in Europe. Grows in damp shady areas. Prefers clay soils.	Hardy plant. Grows in all soils and in any climate.	Very popular hardy plant. Grows in gardens. Commonly used in cooking.	Scented bush common in Mediterranean areas. Likes dry and arid soil.
Bark	Leaves and Flowers	Leaves and flower-heads	Leaves and flower-heads
Choleretic and non-irritant laxative. Important plant for constipation as it does not irritate the intestines. Activates production of bile. Beneficial at all stages of digestion.	Soothing, softening, anti-inflammatory and a laxative. Very useful in the treatment of constipation as it is a very gentle laxative that stimulates the intestines without harming them.	Digestive, carminative, analgesic. Relieves bloating, flatulence and indigestion. Calms feelings of nausea and encourages production of bile by liver.	Choleretic and tonic. Encourages the production of bile, stimulates digestion and the stomach and relieves flatulence.
1 teaspoon to 0.5 litres (0.8 pints) of cold water. Boil for 5 minutes and then infuse for 10. One cup at bedtime.	2 tablespoons to a large bowl of boiling water. Infuse for 2 minutes. Two or three half-bowls per day, between meals.	1 tablespoon to one bowl of boiling water. Infuse for 10 minutes. Half a bowl after meals, lunch time and evening.	15 gm (4.5 ounces) to 1 litre (1.76 pints) of boiling water. Infuse for 10 minutes. One cup after meals, lunch time and evening.

	Burdock *Lappa major* Composaea family	**Silver birch** *Betula alba* Betulaceae family
Origin	Herbaceous plant common in Northern Europe and in America. Grows on plains and on hills up to 1,800 m (6,000 ft).	Attractive tree with silvery bark, very common in Europe. Grows in damp areas.
Part used	Root	Leaves
Effect	Diuretic, cleansing, sudorific, antiseptic. Increases volume of urine and helps body to get rid of toxins that have accumulated. Helps against cellulite.	Diuretic, cleansing and antiseptic. Cleanses body thoroughly. Very effective in treatment of kidney stones, oedema, high blood pressure, cystitis and gout.
Dosage	2 tablespoons of chopped roots to half a litre (0.8 pints) of cold water. Boil for 2 minutes. Three cups a day between meals.	30 chopped leaves to half a litre (0.8 pints) of boiling water. Three cups a day between meals.

Cleansing plants

Butcher's Broom *Ruscus aculeatus* Lilaceae family	Cat's Whiskers *Othosiphon stamineus* Famille des labiées	Pellitory of the wall *Parietaria officinalis* Urticacea family	Dandelion *Taraxacum officinale* Composeae family
Also known as box holly. Small thorny shrub, evergreen, common in Europe. Likes woody areas and chalky soils.	Shrub originally from Java; widely consumed in Europe today.	Herbaceous plant very common in Europe, Northern Africa and Asia.	Commonly found in fields. Its leaves are consumed in salads.
Root	Leaves	Whole plant	Whole plant
Diuretic, sudorific and anti-inflammatory. Very effective in treatment of inflammation of urinary tracts because of its dual anti-inflammatory and diuretic properties. Encourages perspiration.	Cleansing, diuretic. Rapidly increases volume of urine. Gets rid of waste products (urea and uric acid). Excellent purgative, gets rid of water accumulated in tissues (oedema, cellulite).	Diuretic, cleanser, encourages perspiration, refreshing. Helps expel kidney stones, calms attacks of cystitis and relieves oedema by rapidly increasing volume of urine.	Depurative, reduces cholesterol and acts as a stimulant. Acts on the kidneys, liver and bladder. Helps body to get rid of waste products and lowers cholesterol level slightly.
30 gm (9 ounces) to 1 litre (1.76 pints) of cold water. Boil for 5 minutes and infuse for 15. Two cups a day between meals.	2 tablespoons to half a litre (0.8 pints) of boiling water. Infuse for 10 minutes. Up to three cups a day between meals.	30 gm (9 ounces) to 1 litre (1.76 pints) of cold water. Boil for 10 minutes. Two cups a day between meals.	30 gm (9 ounces) of whole plant to 1 litre (1.76 pints) of cold water. Soak for 2 hours then bring to the boil. Drink one cup 10 minutes before each meal.

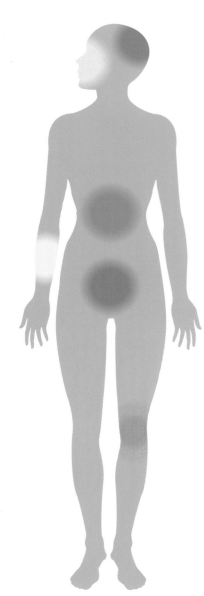

A few indispensable plants

Evening primrose: especially for women
The oil extracted from the seeds is very rich in gammalinolic acid, which increases the level of prostaglandins, resulting in a marked reduction in pre-menstrual symptoms such as irritability and migraines.

Marigold: wonderful healer
Its mother tincture is amazingly effective in speeding up the healing of wounds or burns, thanks to its richness in beta-carotene and flavonoids.

Aloe vera: silky skin
Its gel contains more than 200 active ingredients. It is anti-inflammatory, astringent, healing, an exfoliant and has anti-ageing properties. It is suitable for all types of skin.

Devil's Claw: anti-arthritic
This root from the Kalahari desert is a powerful anti-inflammatory agent which acts on joints. But as digestion often destroys some of its active ingredients it is often taken on the tongue.

Echinacea: for an optimum immune system
Studies have confirmed its stimulating action on the immune system. Its active ingredients, echinachosoids, possess antibiotic properties. It helps to prevent infectious diseases and aids recovery from them. It is sold in capsules, mother tinctures and creams.

Tea-tree: soothing and healing
Its oil has powerful bacterial and fungicide properties, and is effective in treating vaginal infections, skin problems, burns and acne.

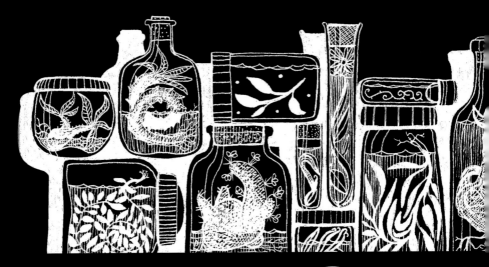

FIND OUT

MORE ABOUT USING PLANTS TO HEAL AND SOOTHE.
THE USES AND PROPERTIES OF BACH'S 38 FLORAL
REMEDIES AND 20 ESSENTIAL OILS.
PLANTS TO CURE EMOTIONAL ILLS.
USEFUL ADDRESSES AND INTERNET SITES.

The Acorn and the Gourd
Jean de La Fontaine, 1671

The extraordinary complexity of plants is not limited to their powers of healing. French poet Jean de la Fontaine illustrated the cleverness of nature through a fable.

All that Jove does is wise and good,
I need not travel far abroad
To make this maxim understood,
But take example from a Gourd.
Observing once a pumpkin,
Of bulk so huge on stem so small,
'What meant he?' cried a bumpkin,
'Great Jove, I mean, who made us all,
By such an act capricious?
If my advice were asked by Heaven,
To yonder oaks the gourds were given,
And 'twould have been judicious;
For sure it is good taste to suit
To monstrous trees a monstrous fruit...
The more I view this sad abortion
Of all the laws of true proportion,
The more I'm sure the Lord of Thunder
Has made a very serious blunder.'
Teased by this matter, Tony cries,
'One soon grows weary when one is wise;'
Then dozing 'neath an oak he lies.
Now, as he slept, an Acorn fell
Straight on his nose, and made it swell.
At once awake, he seeks to trace

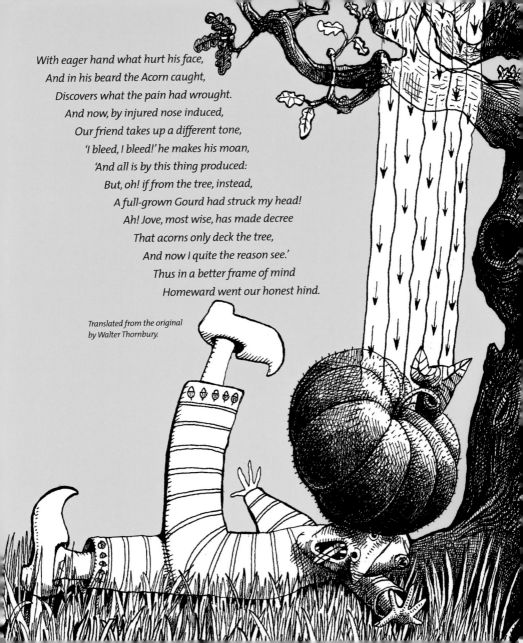

With eager hand what hurt his face,
And in his beard the Acorn caught,
Discovers what the pain had wrought.
And now, by injured nose induced,
Our friend takes up a different tone,
'I bleed, I bleed!' he makes his moan,
'And all is by this thing produced:
But, oh! if from the tree, instead,
A full-grown Gourd had struck my head!
Ah! Jove, most wise, has made decree
That acorns only deck the tree,
And now I quite the reason see.'
Thus in a better frame of mind
Homeward went our honest hind.

Translated from the original
by Walter Thornbury.

The secret language of nature
David Bellamy and Andrea Pfister

David Bellamy, botanist, writer and broadcaster, has become one of the best-known personalities in Britain. Andrea Pfister, a graduate in botany and ecology, works on the human and social aspects of conservation. They took this quotation from an advertisement that appeared in the *International Herald Tribune* and other leading American newspapers in 1990.

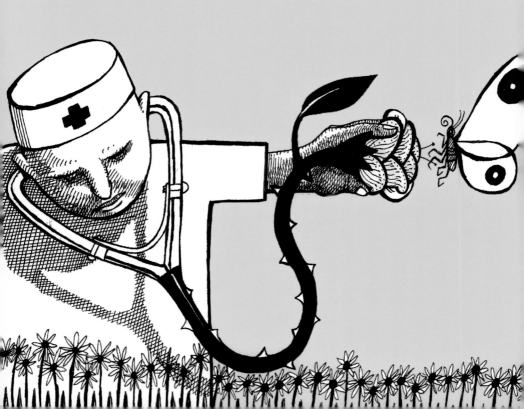

Imagine your fate is entwined with that of a South American vine, or a fragile pink flower in far off Madagascar. If these plants were threatened with extinction, you would spring to their defence.

What if we told you that many patients facing major surgery rely on a muscle relaxant extracted from an Amazonian vine, *Chrondroendron tomentosum*?

Or that four out of five children with leukaemia survive, thanks to the chemicals vincristine and vinblastine, donated by the rosy periwinkle?

Would the fate of these plants raise your concern? If so, read on.

It is essential that you be aroused beyond mere concern, to action...

Extracts from an Amazonian oak tree coagulate proteins, immensely helping scientists in the search for an AIDS vaccine. People sleep deeply and breathe easily during operations thanks to scopolamine derived from mandrake, henbane, and thorn apples. Cancer of the lung, kidney and testis responds to Etoposide, a drug synthesised from May apples...

Women who take the contraceptive pill for granted would not be taking it at all were it not for the yam. This large tuber is the source of the Pill's active ingredient, diosgenin.

Peptic ulcers heal faster thanks to the pale blue petals and flat brown pods of liquorice flower, origin of carbenoxalone.

...Now this vast store of known and potential medicines is under threat and we are all of us obliged to protect it...

Ladies and gentlemen, this is our last chance. The world, our world, is dying from an iatrogenic disease caused by a pathogen called Homo sapiens, which is destroying the life support system of the Earth and the best-stocked pharmacy there has ever been. If the medical profession in all its guises can't see that its way ahead is through a new eclectic, the best of the old with the best of the new working in symbiosis to solve the real problems of this, the saddest of centuries, the future hasn't a chance. We must use the green print of medicare handed down to the West over more than 30,000 years to reach a very attainable and respectable goal: every child a wanted child, growing up into an individual who can aspire to the dignity of a truly civilised world and an average active life of perhaps a little more than three score years and ten, leading on to an active old age, not *sans* eyes, *sans* teeth, *sans* everything, but *sans* pain and the anguish of geriatric syndromes.

David Bellamy and Andrea Pfister

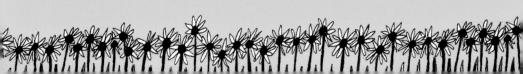

Plants to cure emotional ills

Some doctors have developed original views on plants. French doctor Bernard Vial believes that plants are capable of curing the emotional problems that could be the cause of numerous diseases. An article published in the magazine *Médicine Douce* (Alternative Medicine), July–August 1993 written by Françoise Nahmias, sums up this surprising take on herbalism. Here are a few extracts.

What is emotional medicine?

'Every disease is a state of uneasiness, an inability to express an emotional disorder or the failure of it being understood.' This idea, proposed by Doctor Vial, underpins the logic of 'emotional medicine'. Thus, behind bronchitis is often hidden 'an unhappy family environment' and asthma masks 'a stifled love-song'. Doctor Vial's theory led him to explore the relationships between emotions and disease and the possibility of removing the blockages causing disease with the use of appropriate medicinal plants.

This treatment rests on two hypotheses. On the one hand, a well-targeted plant remedy can change the emotional mood of a patient and can thus help him with his problems. On the other hand, proteins in blood serum provide the biological support for this change. These serum proteins are sensitive to failures and disappointments. They carry the emotional 'scars' of each person. Once the events have been imprinted, these blood molecules transmit the negative information to the organs, the source of psychosomatic symptoms.

By using specific plant remedies that carry new information to the serum proteins, it is possible to target the disturbed emotions and to help them emerge. This information stops the emotional disturbance and diminishes the risks of psychosomatic symptoms. Cured from its 'emotional wound', the protein structure is once again open to other emotions. To benefit from this particular treatment the patient can take the plant in tablet or tincture form, or inhale it.

This medical practice stems from a series of observations and experiments carried out in the field by more than 200 general practitioners in France over a period of 20 years. To date the 'emotional impact' of 1,200 plants has been identified.

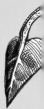

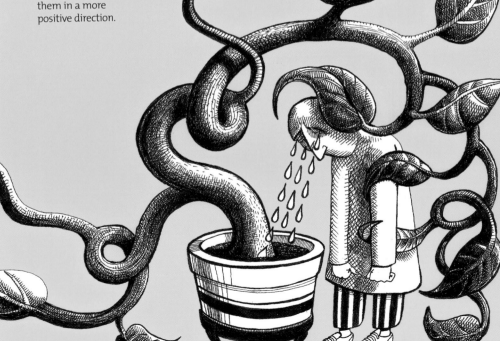

Discover your plant

Bearing in mind the theory of plants helping to cure our emotional ills, select the plants you like best from the following tables. Your choice will speak volumes about your emotional state. You can then read about the strength of your chosen plant to modify your emotions, guiding them in a more positive direction.

FLOWERS

PLANTS	YOU ARE	YOU WILL BECOME
Rose	...rigid, intolerant, cut off from happiness, closed to others.	...generous but very attached to your principles.
Lily	...subject to continuous anguish which paralyses your spontaneity.	...endowed with a subtle sense of humour which will temper your seriousness.
Poppy	...very shy, the eternal adolescent, you feel unable to cope with adult life.	...open to new experiences, open emotionally.
Narcissus	...lacking in self regard.	...indulgent towards others and self-aware.
Periwinkle	...emotionally insecure, verging on arrogance; cynical, you like challenges in order to prove your superiority.	...sure of yourself, without feeling the need for competition with others and yourself.

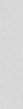

TREES	YOU ARE/HAVE	YOU WILL BECOME
Oak	...difficulties in affirming your autonomy within the family, trapped between insecurity and authority.	...independent, responsible, solid; you will learn how to help others to overcome their problems.
Olive tree	...in the grips of savage resentment, you are merciless in battle.	...clear-headed, thoughtful, kindly and courteous, without excessive familiarity.
Maritime pine	...sensitive to praise and like to be protective.	...courageous, altruistic, with a need to be recognised but still wanting to defend the helpless.
Palm tree	...the feeling of being a superior being, of always being right. You become violent if you are crossed.	...an honest person who has a good mind.
Birch	...found it difficult to recover from the failure of a first love-affair and have renounced sexuality for the intellect.	...endowed with a great understanding of feelings and the heart, without being pedantic.

PLANTS	YOU ARE/HAVE	YOU WILL BECOME
Rubber plant	... a tendency to be hard-hearted through lack of contact with reality.	...attentive towards your friends and see material issues in the right perspective.
Mother-in-law plant	... a feeling of constantly being betrayed or slandered, you oscillate between anger and confusion.	...capable of refusing easy solutions, you will break away from situations which do not suit you.
Begonia	...a perfectionist with confused desires.	...capable of learning from your mistakes and will make commitments in spite of doubts.
Hydrangea	...a prisoner of family quarrels.	...an idealist who refuses the trappings of power.
Geranium	...an agitated mind and unachievable goals.	...independent and courageous, capable of affirming yourself no matter the situation or company.

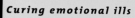

SPICES		
PLANTS	**YOU ARE/HAVE**	**YOU WILL BECOME**
Cinnamon	...the feeling that you are diminished if others are not fulsome in their praise of you.	...modest, love honesty, detest a lack of sincerity.
Nutmeg	...susceptible, infantile in amorous relationships, tyrannical because of your hidden fragility.	...playful and charming, drawing on the world of children to liven up the daily round.
Cloves	...changeable, varying from being inordinately over-confident to totally self-deprecating.	...capable of doing without others' approval and of adapting to any situation.
Pepper	...incapable of expressing your desires for fear of breaking the rules.	...inspired by a deep sense of values and able to make long-term commitments when you are sure of your feelings.
Ginger, curry	...unhealthily shy, you feel the need to feel protected by those around you.	...capable of living your own life whilst managing your nearest and dearest yet you will still be able to dispense with convention if need be.

HERBS		
PLANTS	**YOU ARE/HAVE**	**YOU WILL BECOME**
Borage	...convinced that you must atone for mistakes committed by the people around you.	...capable of looking at others tolerantly and without prejudice.
Clover	...a tendency to lose yourself in daily preoccupations to escape from reality.	...organised, efficient, open, broad-minded.
Lavender	...worn out by an incessant stream of petty family disputes.	...a peacemaker who knows the just measure of things.
Horsetail	...eternally misunderstood, too vulnerable to defend yourself. You have a constant sense of injustice.	...adaptable and capable of taking an objective look at life.
Nettle	...under the impression that you are a victim and remain traumatised by painful emotional experiences.	...warm and ironic, will not let yourself be easily tamed.

A few preconceptions clarified

Much has been said about herbal medicine, some of it contradictory and some false ideas die hard while certain truths are not easily accepted. Here is the low-down on a few common preconceptions.

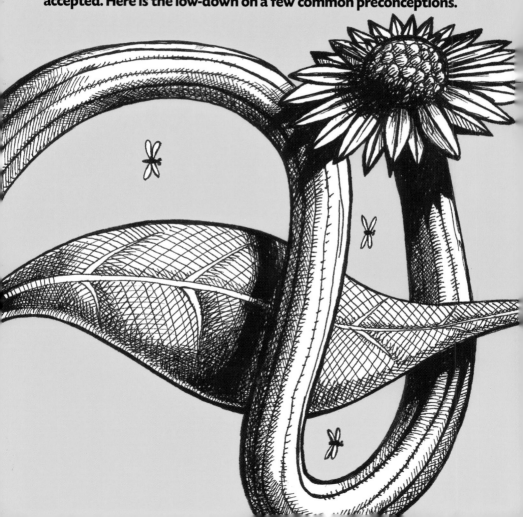

1. Herbalists no longer exist.		5. New methods of administering plants have made them flavour of the month again.	
TRUE	FALSE	TRUE	FALSE
2. Herbal medicine is not a 'soft' option.		**6. Plants are less effective than chemical medicines.**	
TRUE	FALSE	TRUE	FALSE
3. Herbal medicine is an old-fashioned medicine.		**7. All diseases can be cured by plants.**	
TRUE	FALSE	TRUE	FALSE
4. Plants should not be used to treat children and old people.			
TRUE	FALSE		

1. FALSE.

2. TRUE. Although it is a natural medicine it can be toxic and dangerous. This is why it is not advisable to follow a treatment without the advice of a specialist (herbalist, pharmacist, doctor or therapist) and why it is important to follow the directions scrupulously. Even non-toxic plants can cause problems if they are wrongly used, eg. too much liquorice can increase blood pressure and excessive dandelion can drain potassium reserves.

3. FALSE. Herbal medicine is certainly very old – its origins are lost in the proverbial mists of time. However, modern science has confirmed the therapeutic efficacy of plants, in the majority of cases, discovering substances within plants that confirm and explain their traditional uses.

4. FALSE. Plants are suitable for people of all ages. However, it is especially important that children and old people follow carefully the advice of a specialist and do not improvise the dose or treatment. The reason for this is that the negative side effects of certain plants are stronger in the very young and the very old.

5. TRUE. Plants today are packaged in capsules, ampoules and drops that are simpler and easier to use and better adapted to the modern lifestyle.

6. TRUE AND FALSE. Plants provide ingredients for nearly 70 per cent of conventional medicines. Medicinal plants contain active substances that have a direct biological effect on the body, as do conventional medicines. Conventional medicines often contain a single active substance, whereas plants have a more complex structure. Conventional medicines have a more precise and rapid action but are often linked with troubling secondary effects, whereas plants act more slowly but are tolerated better by the body.

7. FALSE. We shouldn't ask too much from plants. They are powerless in curing some serious illnesses (eg cancer, AIDS, auto-immune diseases). However, they do offer useful complementary treatments. Moreover, we mustn't forget that scientists throughout the world are searching the plant world for medicines capable of curing today's incurable diseases.

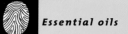

Essential oils

Learn how to use essential oils and extracts of aromatic plants to heal the body and calm the soul, by using floral remedies and flower extracts.

PLANT EXTRACTS		
OIL	**PROPERTIES**	
Basil *(Ocimum basilicum)*	Analgesic, expectorant, tonic.	
Bergamot *(Citrus bergamia)*	Antiseptic, stimulant.	
Bois de rose *(Rosa centifolia)*	Antiseptic, sedative.	
Camomille *(Matricaria)*	Anti-inflammatory, sedative, antispasmodic.	
Cinnamon *(Cinamomum)*	Antiseptic, analgesic, anti-inflammatory, tonic.	
Cumin *(Cuminium cyminum)*	Digestive.	
Eucalyptus *(Eucalyptus globulus)*	Antiseptic, anti-inflammatory, analgesic, expectorant, balsamic.	
Garlic *(Allium sarivum)*	Antiseptic, lowers blood pressure, antiviral.	
Jasmine *(Jasminum officinale)*	Sedative, tonic, moisturising.	
Juniper *(Juniperus communis)*	Antispasmodic, antiseptic, stimulant, carminative, diuretic.	
Lavender *(Lavandula officinalis)*	Antiseptic, tonic, diuretic, astringent.	
Lemon *(Citrus limonum)*	Antiseptic, antiviral, analgesic, sedative.	
Oregano *(Origanum vulgare)*	Antiseptic, antiviral, anti-inflammatory, appetite-stimulant.	
Peppermint *(Mentha piperita)*	Stimulant, analgesic, antiseptic, helps the liver.	
Rosemary *(Rosmarinus officinalis)*	Antiseptic, fungicide, diuretic, stimulant, antidepressant.	
Seville orange *(Citrus aurantium)*	Sedative, hypnotic, antiseptic, lowers blood-pressure.	
Tea tree *(Melaleuca alternifolia)*	Antiseptic, fungicide, antibiotic, antiviral.	
Thyme *(Thymus vulgaris)*	Antiseptic, antiviral, anti-inflammatory, tonic.	
Vervain *(Verbena officinalis)*	Tonic, digestive, antiseptic.	
Ylang-Ylang *(Cananga odorata)*	Sedative, antidepressant, lowers blood-pressure.	

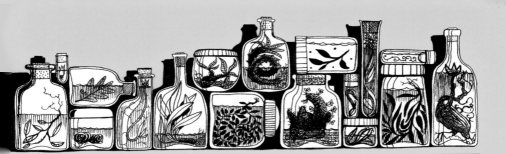

INDICATIONS	HOW TO USE
Fatigue, migraine, colds, coughs, nausea.	Inhalations, oral consumption, massage, baths.
Depression, fatigue, skin problems.	Inhalations, compresses, baths, massage.
Skin problems, wrinkles, stress.	Massage, baths.
Stress, anxiety, insomnia, inflammation, stomach problems.	Compresses, oral consumption, baths.
Infectious diseases, respiratory diseases, fatigue.	Oral consumption, inhalations, massage.
Indigestion, liver problems.	Oral consumption, massage.
Bronchial diseases, herpes, cystitis, rheumatism.	Massage, inhalations, baths
Wounds, high blood-pressure, coughs, colds.	Massage, oral consumption.
Stress, nervousness, depression, dry skin.	Oral consumption, massage, baths.
Liver problems, urinary infections, rheumatism, cellulite.	Baths, oral consumption, massage.
Fatigue, skin problems, infections, warts.	Compresses, baths, gargles, oral consumption, massage.
Burns, skin infections, stress, insomnia, anxiety, headaches.	Massage, baths, oral consumption.
Respiratory problems, viral infections, loss of appetite.	Oral consumption, massage, compresses, baths.
Nausea, headaches, colds, tiredness, emotional shocks.	Oral consumption, inhalations, compresses, massage.
Fatigue, sprains, water retention, rheumatism.	Oral consumption, massage, baths.
Skin problems, stress, insomnia, high blood pressure.	Baths, massage, compresses.
Fungal diseases, thrush, infectious diseases.	Inhalations, compresses, baths, massage.
Infectious diseases, viral illnesses, fatigue, rheumatism.	Oral consumption, inhalations.
Fatigue, indigestion.	Oral consumption, massage.
Stress, nervousness, anxiety, depression, high blood pressure.	Baths, massage, diffusion in atmosphere.

Dr Bach's 38 floral remedies

THE SUBTLETY OF FLOWERS

REMEDY	FLOWER OF ORIGIN	INDICATIONS
Agrimony	Agrimonia eupatoria	Helps those who hide their malaise under an exterior of cheerfulness to regain inner peace and harmony.
Beech	Fagus sylvatica	Quietens intolerant, critical people who believe themselves always in the right.
Centauria	Centaurea	Strengthens the will, reinforces the capacity to assert oneself and to find one's rightful place.
Cerato	Ceratostigma willmottianum	Helps those who find it difficult to take the initiative and rely on others. Helps one to make choices and to carry them through.
Cherry plum	Prunus cerasifera	Helps those who are frightened of losing control of themselves and who feel at the end of their tether.
Chicory	Cichorium intybus	Helps those who are possessive, stubborn or egocentric; helps them to forgive.
Clematis	Clematis vitalba	For those who have their head in the clouds, helps them to focus and live in the present and to carry out their daily tasks.
Common rock rose	Helianthemum nummularium	Remedy for emergencies. To help overcome fear and trauma, to find the courage to act.
Crab apple	Malus pumila	For those who are preoccupied by cleanliness and purity and who make mountains out of molehills.
Dog rose	Rosa canina	Combats lethargy and apathy and brings back a lust for life.
Elm	Ulmus procera	For those who take on important responsibilities but feel that they have bitten off more than they can chew.
Gentian	Gentiana	Combats pessimism and discontent and brings back confidence and will.
Gorse	Ulex europaeus	Helps those who have lost all hope to accept life's difficulties.
Heather	Calluna vulgaris	Curbs the excesses of the ego, brings relaxation and inner calm. Encourages consideration of those around you.
Holly	Ilex aquifolium	A remedy for jealousy, mistrust and suspicion. Awakens sincere love.
Honeysuckle	Lonicera caprifolium	Helps those nostalgic for the past to rediscover the joys of the present and to contemplate the future with serenity.
Hornbeam	Carpinus betulus	Reinforces motivation, revives enthusiasm in cases of mental fatigue. Reinforces capacity for adaptation, gives back a taste for life.
Horse Chestnut bud	Aesculus hippocastanum	Calms irritability, impatience, anger and edginess born of inner tension. Allows one to take one's time to do things properly.
Impatiens	Impatiens	Adjusts self-confidence. Helps one to accept failure more easily, but also to expect disappointment less often. Helps shy and sensitive people who suffer from constant feelings of insecurity and suppressed fear.

MEDY	FLOWER OF ORIGIN	INDICATIONS
ch	Larix decidua	Helps shy and sensitive people who suffer from constant feelings of insecurity and fear.
nkey flower	Mimulus guttatus	Relieves recurrent but short-lived bouts of melancholy, sadness and even deep depression.
stard	Brassica hirta	Helps hard workers and those who shoulder other people's burdens to recharge their batteries and gain a sense of proportion.
k	Quercus robur	Helps those who suffer from non-constructive self-criticism and constant feelings of guilt.
e	Pinus sylvestris	Helps those who are always worried about others, even without reason, and who tend to fear the worst.
d chestnut	Aesculus carnea	Helps to overcome physical and mental shocks and to cope with emergency situations.
scue Remedy	Rock rose, Star of Bethlehem, impatiens, plum and clematis.	Relieves daily feelings of inexpressed insecurity and anxiety, especially in shy and sensitive people.
arlet monkey musk	Mimulus cardinalis	Calms repressed anger and aggression and aids self-assertion. For those who suffer from mood swings and are constantly in a melancholy and doubting frame of mind.
leranthus	Scleranthus anuus	Stabilises them and helps them to make decisions.
ring water	Pure water from protected sources	Helps those who are too strict with themselves to rediscover the pleasures of the senses and feelings; helps with finding inner peace.
ar of Bethlehem	Ornithogalum umbellatum	'Great comforter'. To help recover from physical and mental shocks, recent or old.
veet chestnut	Castanea sativa	Revives hope in moments of extreme anguish and despair.
veet violet	Viola odorata	Remedy for very shy, self-effacing, sensitive people who find it hard to impose themselves and who retreat in order to protect themselves.
ervain	Verbena officinalis	Curbs the optimism of those who always think they are right and want to impose their views on others. Makes people more tolerant and reflective.
ine	Vitis vinifera	Mellows inflexible, proud, over-assertive people and helps them learn to listen and develop respect for others.
Valnut	Juglans regia	'Chain breaker', which helps people break out of old situations and deal with new ones better. Facilitates change.
Vhite chestnut	Aesculus hippocastanum	Calms over-active minds, helping to develop moments of mental relaxation and peace.
ild oat	Bromus ramosus	Helps those who, in spite of their great capabilities, have difficulty in finding their way; helps them to make the right choices and to give free rein to their real qualities.
Villow	Salix	Helps those who bear grudges and who always silently blame others.

Further reading

Frank J. Lipp, *Herbalism*, Duncan Baird, 2000.

Susan Hawkey, *Herbalism*, Southwater, 2000.

Scott Cunningham,*Magical Herbalism: the Secret Craft of the Wise*, Llewellyn Publications, 1985.

Simon Mills, *Modern Herbalism Dictionary: A Comprehensive Guide to Practical Herbal Theory*, 1997.

Frank J. Lipp, *Living Wisdom: Herbalism*, Pan, 1996.

P. Tomkins and C. Bird, *The Secret Life of Plants*, Pocket, 1975.

Paul Beyerl, *The Master Book of Herbalism*, Bookpeople, 1984.

Matthew Wood, *Vitalism: The History of Herbalism, Homeopathy and Flower Essences*, North Atlantic Books, 2000.

Ellen Evert Hopman, *Walking the World in Wonder: A Children's Herbal*, Healing Art Press, 2000.

Non Shaw, *Herbalism: an Illustrated Guide*, Element Books, 1998.

Jerry Stannard, *Herbs and Herbalism in the Middle Ages and Renaissance*, Variorum, 1999.

Julia Lawless, *The Illustrated Encyclopedia of Essential Oils: The Complete Guide to the Use of Oils in Aromatherapy and Herbalism*,Element Books Inc, 1995

Floral remedies

Philip Salmon et al, *Dr Bach's Flower Remedies and the Chakras*, Energy Works.

Dr. Andrew Lockie and Dr. Nicola Geddes, *Homeopathy, principles and treatments*, Reader's Digest, 1996.
An illustrated introduction to homeopathic medicine and its use of plants.

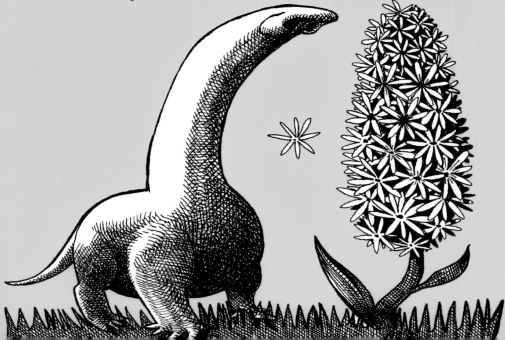

Aromatherapy

Scott Cunningham, *Magical Aromatherapy: the Power of Scent*, Llewellyn Publications, 1989.
A more whimsical look at the magical properties of flowers, oils, spices and their fragrances.

Patricia Davis, Sarah Budd (Illustrator), *Aromatherapy: an A-Z*, Health Science Press, 1988.
A general reference work in an easily accessible format.

Cathy Hopkins, *Principles of Aromatherapy*, HarperCollins, 1996.

Claire Maxwell-Hudson, *OK Living: Aromatherapy Massage*. Dorling Kindersley, 1999.
19 essential oils explained and illustrated; their history, properties, massages and daily uses.

Shirley Price, *Practical Aromatherapy*, HarperCollins, 2000.
A new edition that has chapters on Holism and Swiss Reflex Therapy and includes information on the availability of oils and how to prepare and blend them.

Carol Schiller and David Schiller, *500 Formulas for Aromatherapy*, Sterling Publishing, 1994.
A guide to what treatments can be obtained by blending a range of easily-obtainable essential oils. There are recipes for massage oils, scented candles, beauty treatments and shampoos as well as for minor ailments such as the common cold.

Kurt Schnaubelt, *Advanced Aromatherapy: the Science of Essential Oil Therapy*, Healing Art Press, 1998.
A close look at the effects of essential oils on the human body. A research-based reference work.

Valerie Ann Worwood, *Fragrant Pharmacy*, Bantam, 1991.
From the author of *Aromantics*, a study of the usefulness of essential oils in treating sports injuries, stress-related disorders, in health, beauty, pregnancy and childbirth, cooking and even petcare.

Tibetan medicine

Terry Clifford, *Tibetan Buddhist Medicine and Psychiatry*, Samuel Weiser, 1990.
Makes a good read without taking short cuts. Includes translations of the chapters of the Third Tantra relating to Tibetan psychiatry.

Peter Fenton, *Tibetan Healing: The Modern Legacy of Medicine Buddha*, Quest Books, 1999.
A study of the medicine Buddha tradition that also explores ways in which Western lifestyles may benefit from its teachings.

Elisabeth Finckh, *Studies in Tibetan Medicine*, Snow Lion Publications, 1988

Kenneth Meadows, *The Flight of the Eagle*, Pocket, 1998.
How to follow the Shamanic way, programme organised by a British university using traditional Shaman methods.

Tamdin Sither Bradley, *Principles of Tibetan Medicine*, HarperCollins, 2000.
Takes a hands on approach, describing exercises and a range or treatments that can be made with widely-available herbs. Also includes an international resource directory and some useful case histories.

Chinese medicine

Complete Chinese Medicine, Mustard, 1999.

Harriet Beinfield, Efrem Korngold, *Between Heaven and Earth : A Guide to Chinese Medicine*, Ballantine Books, 1992.
Looks at Chinese medicine, its different treatment methods and the philosophy behind it.

Duo Gao and Dr Duo, *The Encyclopedia of Chinese Medicine*, Carlton Books, 2000

Letha Hadady, *Asian Health Secrets : The Complete Guide to Asian Herbal Medicine*, Crown Publishing Group, 1998.
A book that looks at the practical side of Chinese medicine, with guides to self-diagnosis and treatment with readily available herbs.

David Molony and others, *The American Association of Oriental Medicine's Complete Guide to Chinese Herbal Medicine*, Berkley Publishing Group, 1998.
A thorough study that places Chinese medicine in its historical context and describes herbal treatments in detail. It also explores the relevance of the ying/yang concept to medicinal treatments.

Anna Selby, *The Ancient and Healing Art of Chinese Herbalism*, Hamlyn, 1998.

Ron Teeguarden, *Chinese Tonic Herbs*, Japan Publications, 1985.
A guide to life-enhancing Chinese herbal treatments.

Associations

SPECIALISTS

SCHOOL OF HERBAL MEDICINE/ PHYTOTHERAPY
Bucksteep Manor
Bodle Street Green
Near Hailsham
Sussex BN27 4RJ
Tel: 01323 833812
Fax: 01323 833869

NATIONAL INSTITUTE OF MEDICAL HERBALISTS
56 Longbrook Street
Exeter
Devon EX4 6AH
Tel: 01392 426022
Fax: 01392 498963

GENERAL COUNCIL AND REGISTER OF CONSULTANT HERBALISTS
18 Sussex Square
Brighton BN2 5AA
Tel: 01243 267126

BRITISH HOMEOPATHIC ASSOCIATION
27a Devonshire Street
London W1N 1RJ
Tel: 020 7935 2163

AMERICAN HERBALISTS GUILD
PO Box 1683
Soquel
California 95073
USA
Tel: 001 831 427 1017

Environment

WWF (WORLD WIDE FUND FOR NATURE)
The most important international organisation for the protection of nature which, amongst other things, protects threatened natural species, especially plants. The WWF websites keep people informed with news, practical actions and current projects.

WWF-UK
Panda House
Weyside Park
Godalming
Surrey GU7 1XR
Tel: 01483 426444
Fax: 01483 426409

GREENPEACE
The most militant of the associations for the protection of the environment, especially for the protection of plants.

GREENPEACE UK
Canonbury Villas
London N1 2PN
Tel: 020 7865 8100
Fax: 020 7865 8200
E-mail:
info@uk.greenpeace.org

Training

RESEARCH AND TRAINING ON FLORAL REMEDIES

EDWARD BACH CENTRE
Research centre created by Edward Bach himself which is still very active.

Mount Vernon
Sotwell
Wallingford
Oxon OX10 0PZ
Tel: 01491 834678
Email:
mail@bachcentre.com
Web site:
www.bachcentre.com

SEMINAR PROGRAMME

BACH FLOWER REMEDIES
Workshops and seminars led by qualified trainers from the Bach Foundation.

Broadheath House
83 Parkside
Wimbledon
London SW19 5LP
Tel: 020 8780 4200

Internet

INTERNATIONAL REGISTER OF CONSULTANT HERBALISTS
www.irch.org

WORLD HEALTH ORGANISATION
www.who.int

HERBAL AND ALTERNATIVE MEDICINE AVAILABLE ON THE INTERNET
www.herbalmed.co.uk

THE GARDEN PHARMACY
The UK's largest online perfumery and pharmacy.

www.garden.co.uk
www.goodnessdirect.co.uk
www.thinknatural.com
www.herbalnet.co.uk
www.health4all.co.uk

NATIVE AMERICAN MEDICAL PLANTS DATABASE
Index of 2,147 plants and their uses.

www.healthfinder.gov/
text/docs/Doc3709.htm

REGISTER OF QUALIFIED AROMATHERAPISTS.
You can search for an aromatherapist in your local area, or read about aromatherapy's aims and objectives and what is involved in obtaining a qualification.

www.rqa-uk.org

BRITISH COMPLEMENTARY MEDICINE ASSOCIATION
Keeps a register of affiliated organisations, including teaching institutions, and helps you find a local therapist.

www.bcma.co.uk

BRITISH HERBAL MEDICINE ASSOCIATION
Founded in 1964 with the aim of advancing the interests of those interested in using and producing herbal medecines.
Publishes British Herbal Pharmacoepia.

www.ex.ac.uk/phytonet/
bhma.html

BRITISH HOMEOPATHIC ASSOCIAION.
Founded in 1902 to promote education and research in homeopathy. Will help you find homeopathic treatment on the NHS. The Faculty of Homeopathy carries out research and trains homeopathic health professionals.

www.trusthomeopathy.
org

REGISTER OF CHINESE HERBAL MEDICINE
Represents UK-based Chinese herbalists.

www.rchm.co.uk

CURRENT RESEARCH

CLINICAL RESEARCH ON MEDICAL PLANTS USED IN HIV INFECTION
Review of clinical studies of the use of medicinal plants in the treatment of AIDS patients.

www.exodus.it/poiesis/
ENG/report/clinical.html

EUROPEAN SCIENTIFIC COOPERATIVE ON PHYTOTHERAPY
Co-ordinates research and regulation of herbal medicine in European countries – a forum for discussion for national herbal medicine associations.

www.escop.com

NATIONAL CENTER FOR COMPLEMENTARY AND ALTERNATIVE MEDICINE
A department of the National Institutes of Health in the USA, the NCCAM is involved in investigation and research in alternative medicine treatments.

http://nccam.nih.gov

HEALING WITH PLANTS

ALMAROME
A site specialising in natural medicines and especially herbalism and essential oils. General and practical information and an online shop where you can buy plants and essential oils.

www.almarome.com

DOCUMENTATION

MEDITERRANEAN INSTITUTE OF DOCUMENTATION AND RESEARCH ON MEDICINAL PLANTS
A newsletter, news, courses at the Institute, calendar of events.

www.imderplam.net

INTERNET RESOURCES

INTERNET HEALTH LIBRARY
News, information and links, updated daily.

www.internethealthlibrary
.com

QUEST HEALTH LIBRARY
Deals with health issues, diet, homeopathic and herbal treatments. Includes links, news items and an index of useful herbs.

www.questhealthlibrary
.com

Glossary

ACIDIC
Describes plants that are mildly acidic and used to ease thirst.

ALCHEMY
Science dating from the Middle Ages. Precursor of modern chemistry, with a touch of magic. Alchemists searched in particular for the universal remedy which would cure all ills and tried to find a formula for changing base metal into gold.

ANALEPTIC
Describes plants that give strength back to patients and convalescents.

ANALGESIC
Describes plants that relieve pain.

ANTIBIOTIC
Used to treat bacterial infection.

ANTIDIURETIC
Diminishes the production of urine.

ANTICOAGULANT
Diminishes the coagulant properties of blood.

ANTI-INFLAMATORY
Used to calm and reduce inflammation

ANTISEPTIC
Describes plants that prevent the proliferation of germs (e.g. bacteria and viruses.)

ANTISPASMODIC
Reduces muscle spasm and tension.

ANTISUDORIFIC
Describes plants that reduce perspiration.

ANTIVIRAL
Acts against viral infection

APERITIF
Describes plants that stimulate the appetite.

APHRODISIAC
Plants that excite the senses, increase desire and stimulate sexual activity.

AROMATHERAPY
Branch of herbalism that consists of the therapeutic use of essential oils.

AROMATIC
Plants that contain strong flavours and scents, and from which essential oils are distilled.

ASTRINGENT
Plants which tighten tissue, especially blood vessels.

AYURVEDIC (MEDICINE)
Traditional medicine of ancient India. Based on a collection of traditional philosophical and religious texts, known as vedas.

BALSAMIC
Describes plants that stimulate the respiratory paths.

BECHIC
Describes plants that soothe coughs.

BILE
Brownish-yellow, bitter fluid secreted by the liver to aid digestion.

CARMINATIVE
Describes plants that relieve flatulence.

CHOLAGOGUE
Describes plants that stimulate the secretion of bile.

CHOLERETIC
Describes plants that stimulate the production of bile in the liver.

CORDIAL
Describes plants that stimulate the activity of the heart and the stomach.

DECOCTION
The liquor resulting from boiling plants to extract their essence.

DEPURATIVE
Substance used to counteract impurities.

DIGESTIVE
Used to aid and improve digestion.

DILUTION
Mixing plant extracts with a neutral support such as water or alcohol to modify their effect.

DISTILLATION
Main method of creating essential oils. The plants are heated, and the steam they give off is passed through a still so the essence of the plant can be collected.

DIURETIC
Describes plants that increase the volume of urine and facilitate its evacuation.

EMETIC
Describes plants that induce vomiting.

ENFLEURAGE
Method used to collect essential oils from flowers. The flowers are laid on a layer of wax and the oils are then distilled.

ESSENTIAL OILS
Oily extract of aromatic plants, very rich in active principles (up to 100 times more than in the original plant).

EXPECTORANT

used to describe plants that encourage the coughing up of bronchial secretions that have accumulated in the lungs.

EXPRESSION

A technique used to collect essential oils from citrus fruits consisting of pressing the skin of citrus fruit where the essences are concentrated in small sack-like pockets.

EXTRACTION PHYTOTHERAPY

Branch of phytotherapy that consists of extracting active ingredients from plants and packaging them in the same way as chemical medicines.

FEBRIFUGE

Used to describe plants that lower temperature.

FLORAL REMEDY

Subtle floral extract containing an 'energetic' message. Floral extracts are used to harmonise emotions and states of mind.

FUNGICIDE

Fungus-destroying substance.

GALACTOGOGUE

Describes plants that encourage the secretion of breast milk.

GALENIC

Name given to the packaging of remedies: creams, capsules, drops, extracts and suppositories deriving from the Greek doctor Claudius Galenus.

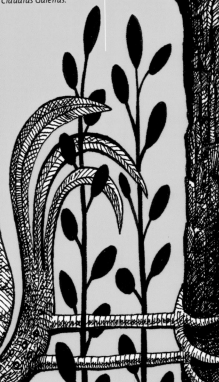

Glossary

HAEMOSTATIC

Describes plants that stop bleeding and haemorrhaging.

HEMISYNTHESIS

Manipulation which consists of isolating molecules containing active principles, then transforming their structure to modify their effects.

HEPATIC

Describes plants that stimulate the functions of the liver.

HYPNOTIC

Describes plants that encourage sleep.

HYPOGLYCAEMIC

Lowers the level of glucose (sugar) in the blood. Hypoglycaemic plants are used especially to treat diabetes.

HYPOLIPIDEMIC

Lowers the level of lipids (fats) in the blood. Hypolipidemic plants are used particularly to combat an excess of cholesterol.

IATROGENIC

(Of disease) resulting unintentionally from medical examination or treatment.

INNOCUOUS

Describes medical treatment (especially using plants) that presents no danger to the patient.

IN VITRO

Describes studies conducted on cells alone and not on complete subjects (such as plants, animals, humans).

IN VIVO

Describes studies on whole living organisms such as plants, animals and humans.

IRRADIATION

Practice that consists of passing plants under gamma rays to stop the proliferation of germs and to preserve them better.

LAXATIVE

Tending to cause evacuation of the bowels.

MACERATION

Softening herbs or roots by soaking in liquid.

OEDEMA

Tissue swollen with fluid.

PATHOLOGY

Part of medicine that determines the causes and forecasts the evolution of diseases.

PERILINGUAL

Describes all remedies that are absorbed by letting them melt on the tongue. The strong presence of blood vessels in the tongue facilitates the absorption of the most fragile active substances into the blood stream through the fine walls of the blood vessels, without being changed by the process of digestion.

PHARMACOPOEIA

A book containing a list of drugs with directions for their use.

PHYTOCHEMISTRY

Branch of herbalism that consists of extracting active substances from plants and studying their chemical structure to find molecules that could be effective in medicines.

PHYTOTHERAPY

Scientific name for herbal medicine. The term comes from the Greek 'phyton', meaning plant, and 'therepeuein' meaning to heal.

PROPHYLATIC

Describes methods that prevent illnesses developing.

PSYCHOSOMATIC

Disease caused or aggravated by mental stress.

PURGATIVE

Describes plants that facilitate the evacuation of metabolic waste and toxins.

RESPIRATORY

Describes remedies which are absorbed by respiration; the active principles pass into the blood at the same time as oxygen through the fine walls of the lungs.

SEDATIVE

Describes plants that calm nervousness, anguish and anxiety.

SHAMAN

Priest or witch doctor claiming to have sole contact with the gods.

SIDE EFFECTS

Secondary, usually undesirable, effects.

SOOTHING

Describes plants that relieve inflammation

SOPORIFIC

Sleep-inducing.

STERNUTATORY

Describes plants that induce sneezing.

STIMULATING

Describes plants that stimulate the nervous system.

STOMACHIC

Used to describe plants that stimulate stomach activity.

SUDORIFIC

Describes plants that increase perspiration.

SULPHONAMIDES

Used to prevent multiplication of some disease-producing bacteria.

SYNERGY

Combined action of different active substances contained in the same plant. Synergy sometimes creates properties that cannot be ascribed to any one particular active principle, but is a product of the collective action.

TANNINS

Substances contained in numerous plants that render them more resistant. Tannins have therapeutic properties.

THERAPEUTIC

Part of medicine that deals with the curing of diseases as opposed to other branches such as diagnosis, for example.

TINCTURE

Method of extraction consisting of macerating plants in alcohol in order to extract substances which are soluble in alcohol.

TITRAGE

A titrated extract is a plant extract that always has the same level of active substances. Titrage is the practice of obtaining this stability, non-existent in the natural state.

TONIC

Restoring, nourishing and supporting for the entire body.

TOTUM

Indicates the use of the whole plant (or the whole of part of a plant) as opposed to the extraction of active substances.

TRANSCUTANEOUS

Used to describe remedies that are applied to the skin. The active substances pass into the bloodstream through the skin.

VERMIFUGE

Describes plants that help to get rid of intestinal worms.

VITALITY

This is the particular character of individuals where health is concerned. It describes the way that individuals react to illnesses with their weak points and strengths. Certain medical practices such as acupuncture and herbalism are called 'vitality medicines' because they try to adapt the treatment to the individual rather than to the illness in general.

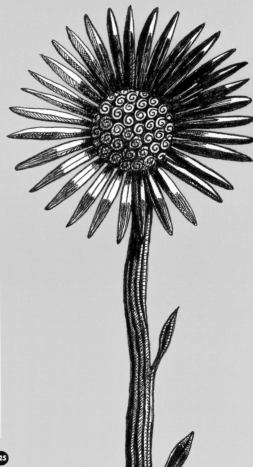

Contents

Fact ⟫ 2–12
Fun facts and quick quotes

Discover ⟫ 13–48

The changing face of Western herbalism   15
Medicinal plants   15
The complexity of living plants and their contribution to health   17
Strong plants and gentle plants   17
When did man first start using plants for medicinal purposes?   19
Lessons to be drawn from Egyptian papyri   19
Hippocrates and Galen: precursors of modern medicine   20
Ancient China: the energy signatures of plants   23
Subtle interplay: how to find a plant capable of restoring the energy balance   25
A bridge between East and West   26
The Ayurvedic tradition: preventative and curative practices still widely used in India   28
Medicine from the roof of the world   31
Shamanism: the spirit of plants   33
Meanwhile in Europe...   34
Paracelsus and the theory of signatures   36
Hahnemann's great discovery   36
From homeopathy to anthroposophy   39
Steiner's theory   40
Edward Bach: the subtle essence of flowers   43
Silent conversations   44
Western medicines derived from tropical forests   44
The amazing creativity of nature   47
Medicines of tomorrow   48

Look ⟫ 49–70

Following the footsteps of the Shamans

In practice ⟫ 71–102

The whole plant 72–73
Traditional uses 74–75
The beneficial effects of tea 76–77
Modern methods of presentation 78–79
Antistress plants 80–81
St John's wort: a plant to combat depression 82–83
With the blessing of science 84–85
The lungs of the planet 86–87
Essential oils: plant concentrates 88–89
How to use essential oils 90–91
Massage using essential oils 92–93
Plants for bronchial problems 94–95
Plants which aid circulation 96–97
Plants that aid digestion 98–99
Cleansing plants 100–101
A few indispensable plants 102

Find out ⟫ 103–125

The Acorn and the Gourd 104–105
The secret language of nature 106–107
Plants to cure emotional ills 108–111
A few preconceptions clarified 112–113
Essential oils – chart 114–115
Dr. Bach's 38 floral remedies 116–117
Further reading 118–119
Addresses and websites 120–121
Glossary 122–125

Picture credits

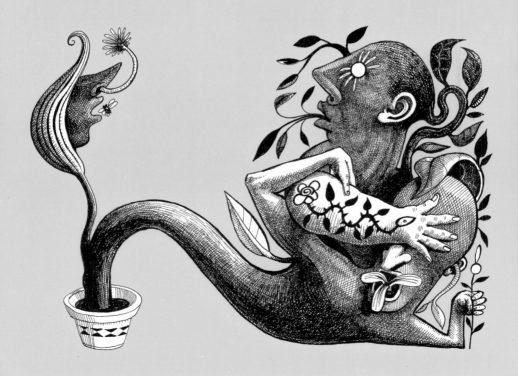